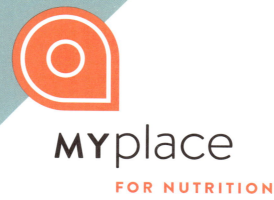

Published by First Place for Health
Galveston, Texas, USA
www.firstplaceforhealth.com
Printed in the USA
© 2018 First Place for Health

Cover design by Faceout Studio, Tim Green
Interior text design by Faceout Studio, Amanda Kreutzer

ISBN 978-1-942425-24-3

Caution: The information contained in this book is intended to be solely for informational and educational purposes. It is assumed that the First Place for Health participant will consult a medical or health professional before beginning this or any other weight-loss or physical fitness program.

It is illegal to copy any part of this document without permission of First Place for Health.

To order copies of this book and other First Place for Health products in bulk quantities, please contact us at 800.727.5223 or on our website: www.firstplaceforhealth.com

All Scripture quotations, unless otherwise indicated, are taken from the Holy Bible, New International Version®, NIV®. Copyright © 1973, 1978, 1984, by Biblica, IncTM. Used by permission of Zondervan Publishing House. All rights reserved worldwide.

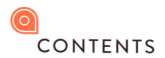

CONTENTS

SECTION 1: THE LIVE-IT FOOD PLAN

Introduction 5
About the Author 9
Choosing a Calorie Level 10
FP4H Food Groups 12
Calorie Information for all Food Groups 16
Using Your Live It Tracker 58

SECTION 2: PRIMARY SESSION WELLNESS WORKSHEETS

Practicing Mindfulness 64
Keeping a Food & Exercise Journal 67
Eating Healthy When Eating Out 71
Understanding Nutrition Labels 76
Recipe Transformation Tactics 83
Habits for a Healthy Heart 88
The Facts on Healthy Fats 93
Preventing and Managing Diabetes 95
Join the Superfoods Fan Club 104

SECTION 3: SUPPLEMENTAL WELLNESS WORKSHEETS

Fiber & Gluten Facts 110
Live It the Vegetarian Way 114
Outsmarting the Snack Attack 117
Preventing Osteoporosis 119
Dieting Dangers & Supplements 123
Weight Loss Maintenance 126

Endnotes 128

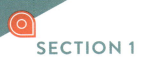

SECTION 1

The Live-It Food Plan

"So whether you eat or drink or whatever you do, do it all for the glory of God."

—1 Corinthians 10:31, NIV

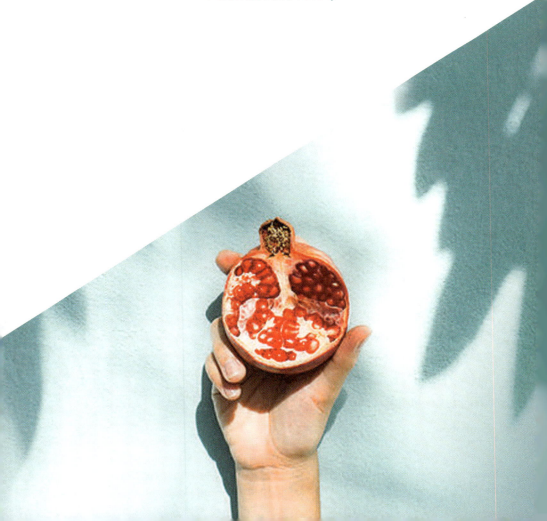

Introduction

Welcome to First Place for Health and a new way of eating for a lifetime!

Some of you are very nervous—or even scared—at this point. You may be thinking, What are they going to make me eat? or Will I be able to understand this? Nutrition is so complicated! Others of you are excited and anxious to get going, having started (and stopped) multiple weight-loss diets in the past. Therefore, you are probably thinking, Just tell me what to do, and I'll do it! Still others of you may have acquired a wealth of good nutrition information and education over the years, so you basically know what you are going to read in the pages ahead—but you aren't currently acting on that knowledge.

When I started leading a First Place for Health (FP4H) group in the spring of 1995, I fell into that last category. As a registered, licensed dietitian, I pretty much knew what (and how much) I should be eating to be healthy. After all, I had spent many hours in nutrition and science classes at Ouachita Baptist University as well as in my dietetic internship at the University of Arkansas for Medical Sciences. I had worked as a clinical dietitian in a hospital, counseling patients about how they should eat. Yet, as a young-adult wife and mother, I had not allowed God to have control over my own eating habits and found myself over 30 pounds overweight. I knew the health risks of that condition and was determined to lose the weight. "I can surely handle that"—or so I thought. After multiple attempts to fix myself, it became very obvious that I couldn't do it alone. Through FP4H, I learned that God wants to be first in every area of my life, including helping me choose and control the foods I put into my mouth. I also learned that I needed (and still need) the accountability of my FP4H group and keeping an actual record of the food I eat to maintain a healthy weight. God used this program to change my life and priorities forever, and He wants to do that for you, too!

One of my favorite parts of the FP4H orientation video back in 1995 was when Kay Smith, associate director of the program at that time, began a discussion of the Live It food plan. She talked about all of the diets she had tried in the past and then asked, "What are the first three letters of that word? That's right—D-I-E! And that's what I felt like I was doing every time I went on one!"

I am very happy to report that the First Place for Health food plan is not a diet—a term that, in the minds of most people, implies a designated beginning and ending time. It also implies boring repetition of the same foods over and over. The Live It food plan is designed to be something you can live with every day for the rest of your life. I can attest to its credibility and success after seeing it work for literally hundreds of my group members and having been on the FP4H program personally for over 20 years.

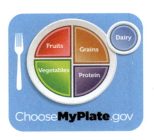

The Live It food plan is based on solid, scientific, research-based nutrition information. So you don't have to worry about it being dangerous or hazardous to you in any way, unlike some of the wacky fad diets that are floating around out there! The foundation of the plan is the United States Department of Agriculture (USDA) and Health and Human Services (HHS) Dietary Guidelines for Americans. "Choose MyPlate," a nutrition education program that expands on these guidelines to help provide specific individual nutrition goals, has become a familiar term in our country.

Every five years, USDA and HHS publish the Dietary Guidelines to reflect the current body of scientific evidence on nutrition, food and health. Their focus is on disease prevention and health promotion. The following 2015-2020 Dietary Guidelines will be the current policy until the release of the next edition in 2020:

1. **Follow a healthy eating pattern across the lifespan.** All food and beverage choices matter. Choose a healthy eating pattern at an appropriate calorie level to help achieve and maintain a healthy body weight, support nutrient adequacy, and reduce the risk of chronic disease.

2. **Focus on variety, nutrient density, and amount.** To meet nutrient needs within calorie limits, choose a variety of nutrient-dense foods across and within all food groups in recommended amounts.

SECTION 1 THE LIVE-IT FOOD PLAN

3. **Limit calories from added sugars and saturated fats, and reduce sodium intake.** Consume an eating pattern low in added sugars, saturated fats, and sodium. Cut back on foods and beverages higher in these components to amounts that fit within healthy eating patterns.

4. **Shift to healthier food and beverage choices.** Choose nutrient-dense foods and beverages across and within all food groups in place of less healthy choices. Consider cultural and personal preferences to make these shifts easier to accomplish and maintain.

5. **Support healthy eating patterns for all.** Everyone has a role in helping to create and support healthy eating patterns in multiple settings nationwide, from home to school to work to communities.

A HEALTHY EATING PATTERN INCLUDES:

A variety of vegetables from all of the subgroups (dark green, red/orange, legumes, starchy, and other)

Fruits, especially whole fruits

Grains, at least half of which are whole grains

Fat-free or low-fat dairy, including milk, yogurt, cheese, and/or fortified soy beverages

A variety of protein foods, including seafood, lean meats and poultry, eggs, legumes (beans and peas), nuts, seeds, and soy productsOils

A HEALTHY EATING PATTERN LIMITS:

Saturated and trans fats, added sugars, and sodium.*

*http://health.gov/dietaryguidelines/2015/guidelines/executive-summary

In summary, the FP4H food plan is balanced, healthy, common sense, and do-able. You don't have to buy special, expensive, prepackaged foods or nutrition supplements from a certain company. There are also no taboo foods (no food is inherently evil; it's just food!), but there are definitely choices that are better for you than others, which you will see in the pages to come. Your goal is to create and sustain a lifestyle of healthy food choices overall, saving room for occasional less-healthy treats but *not* giving them a prominent place in your daily eating pattern.

We also call it the "Live It" because God provides abundant life through Jesus, His Son. We can choose to honor God and even *worship* Him through making healthy food choices for our bodies, His temple:

> *Do you not know that your bodies are temples of the Holy Spirit, who is in you, whom you have received from God? You are not your own; you were bought at a price. Therefore honor God with your bodies.*
>
> —1 Corinthians 6:19-20

Now, I hope you are as excited to learn about the program as I am about sharing it with you. Let the lifelong healthy adventure begin!

SECTION 1 THE LIVE-IT FOOD PLAN

ABOUT THE AUTHOR

Charlotte Davis has led First Place 4 Health groups in Arkansas churches since 1995 and says that she never plans to stop because God forever changed her life and her priorities through the program! She has served as Arkansas Networking Leader for over 15 years and has also served as a speaker (and sometimes Worship Leader) for many national FP4H events including Summit and Wellness Week. Charlotte is a Registered, Licensed Dietitian, is credentialed as a School Nutrition Specialist, and works as the Child Nutrition Director for an Arkansas public school district of about 4100 students. She has been married to Tony Davis since 1987 and they have two grown children (Kayla and Jake). Her favorite activities include spending time/traveling with her family, serving on the Praise and Worship Team in her church, reading Christian literature, cooking, and creating stamped greeting cards to send to her FP4H friends/family.

MYplace O FOR NUTRITION

CHOOSING A CALORIE LEVEL

Calories are the energy in the foods and beverages you consume. They provide the fuel that powers your body. The key to achieving and maintaining a healthy weight lies in calorie balance. Weight *gain* occurs when you take in more calories than your body needs. Similarly, to *lose* weight you must reduce the number of calories you take in (by adjusting your dietary intake) or increase the number of calories you use up (by increasing your level of physical activity), or both.

One pound of weight is equal to 3,500 calories. Therefore, in order to lose a pound a week, you must reduce your daily intake by an average of 500 calories (7 days per week x 500 calories per day), increase your physical activity to *burn* 500 calories a day, or combine the two to reach your goal. To lose two pounds per week (the recommended maximum average weekly weight-loss level), you would need to create a daily deficit of 1,000 calories.

There are various methods for estimating an individual's calorie needs. Personal variables, such as height, weight, age, sex, and activity level, all play a role in tailoring the estimation to you specifically. It is important to remember that most methods provide only an estimate, not an exact determination of calorie needs. See the charts below to assist you with determining a calorie level to follow in FP4H.

Recommended Calorie Ranges for Weigh Loss for Adult Women

AGE	ACTIVITY LEVEL 1* (CALORIES PER DAY)	ACTIVITY LEVEL 2** (CALORIES PER DAY)	ACTIVITY LEVEL 3*** (CALORIES PER DAY)
19-20	1700-1800	1900-2000	2100-2200
21-25	1700-1800	1900-2000	2100-2200
26-30	1500-1600	1700-1800	2100-2200
31-35	1500-1600	1700-1800	1900-2000
36-40	1500-1600	1700-1800	1900-2000
41-45	1500-1600	1700-1800	1900-2000
46-50	1500-1600	1700-1800	1900-2000
51-55	1300-1400	1500-1600	1900-2000
56-60	1300-1400	1500-1600	1900-2000
61-65	1300-1400	1500-1600	1700-1800
66-70	1300-1400	1500-1600	1700-1800
71-75	1300-1400	1500-1600	1700-1800
76+	1300-1400	1500-1600	1700-1800

SECTION 1 **THE LIVE-IT FOOD PLAN**

Recommended Calorie Ranges for Weigh Loss for Adult Men

AGE	ACTIVITY LEVEL 1* (CALORIES PER DAY)	ACTIVITY LEVEL 2** (CALORIES PER DAY)	ACTIVITY LEVEL 3*** (CALORIES PER DAY)
19-20	2200-2400	2400-2600	2600-2800
21-25	2000-2200	2400-2600	2600-2800
26-30	2000-2200	2200-2400	2600-2800
31-35	2000-2200	2200-2400	2600-2800
36-40	2000-2200	2200-2400	2400-2600
41-45	1800-2000	2200-2400	2400-2600
46-50	1800-2000	2000-2200	2400-2600
51-55	1800-2000	2000-2200	2400-2600
56-60	1800-2000	2000-2200	2200-2400
61-65	1600-1800	2000-2200	2200-2400
66-70	1600-1800	1800-2000	2200-2400
71-75	1600-1800	1800-2000	2200-2400
76+	1600-1800	1800-2000	2000-2200

* Activity Level 1 = 1 to 30 minutes of moderate physical activity a day in addition to daily activities.
** Activity Level 2 = 30 to 60 minutes of moderate physical activity a day in addition to daily activities.
*** Activity Level 3 = More than 60 minutes of moderate physical activity a day in addition to daily activities.
If you'd like to maintain your weight, add 200 calories to both end of your range.

Scientific research has shown that it is best to lose weight *slowly*, at a rate of one to two pounds per week. If you decide on a certain calorie level to begin with on FP4H but you find that you are not losing at that rate when consuming all of the food groups recommended in the correct amounts, then you might consider dropping down to the calorie level below (or significantly increasing your activity level). On the other hand, if you are losing *more* than two pounds per week after the initial 2-3 week period on the calorie level (again, making sure that you are consuming all of the food groups in the correct amounts), then you probably need to consider moving up to the calorie level above.

MYplace O FOR NUTRITION

Recommended Daily Amount of Food from Each Group

GROUP	DAILY CALORIES		
....	1300-1400	1500-1600	1700-1800
Fruits	1.5 – 2 c.	1.5 – 2 c.	1.5 – 2 c.
Vegetables	1.5 – 2 c.	2 – 2.5 c.	2.5 – 3 c.
Grains	5 oz.-eq.	5-6 oz.-eq.	6-7 oz.-eq.
Dairy	2-3 c.	3 c.	3 c.
Protein	4 oz.-eq.	5 oz.-eq.	5-5.5 oz.-eq.
Healthy Oils & Other Fats	4 tsp.	5 tsp.	5 tsp.
Water & Super Beverages*	Women: 9 c. Men: 13 c.	Women: 9 c. Men: 13 c.	Women: 9 c. Men: 13 c.

*May count up to 3 cups caffeinated tea or coffee toward goal

THE FIRST PLACE FOR HEALTH FOOD GROUPS

The USDA food guidance system provides suggested amounts of food to consume from the five basic food groups, and oils, to achieve adequate nutrition at several calorie levels. It is important to include *all* of the food groups in any daily eating plan to assure that all of your nutrition needs are met, since each group provides unique nutrients. FP4H has adapted these plans slightly to better reflect our recommendations.

While it is true that you must consume fewer calories than you burn off through activity to have success with losing weight, the calories you take in should contribute not only to weight loss/maintenance but also to health enhancement. First

SECTION 1 THE LIVE-IT FOOD PLAN

1900-2000	2100-2200	2300-2400	2500-2600	2700-2800
2 – 2.5 c.	2 – 2.5 c.	2.5 – 3.5 c.	3.5 – 4.5 c.	3.5 – 4.5 c.
2.5 – 3 c.	3 – 3.5 c.	3.5 – 4.5 c.	4.5 – 5 c.	4.5 – 5 c.
6-7 oz.-eq.	7-8 oz.-eq.	8-9 oz.-eq.	9-10 oz.-eq.	10-11 oz.-eq.
3 c.	3 c.	3 c.	3 c.	3 c.
5.5-6.5 oz.-eq.	6.5-7 oz.-eq.	7-7.5 oz.-eq.	7-7.5 oz.-eq.	7.5-8 oz.-eq.
6 tsp.	6 tsp.	7 tsp.	8 tsp.	8 tsp.
Women: 9 c. Men: 13 c.	Women: 9 c. Men: 13 c.	Women: 9 c. Men: 13 c.	Women: 9 c. Men: 13 c.	Women: 9 c. Men: 13 c.

Place for Health does *not* want to just teach you how to continue eating poorly while losing weight, which may be how you may have lost weight in the past. Just counting calories (or "points") without any consideration of the nutritional value of the foods is not wise. You would not knowingly put trashy gasoline into your car expecting it to perform at its best, would you? In the same manner, if you want your body, God's temple, to function at peak performance, you want to choose the highest quality "fuel" on the market!

Therefore, we have chosen to assist you with making the *best* possible choices in each food group, based on up-to-date nutrition research. Each FP4H food group is divided into three sections: (1) superfoods, (2) everyday foods, and (3) caution foods.

Superfoods: *Foods with Extra Benefits*

The foods in these lists are "premium fuel" choices for your health! They are "super" because they offer health benefits beyond the basics of furnishing energy to your body and should be included as often as possible to create a disease-fighting lifestyle, based on the latest nutrition research. The vast majority of them are what many people call *clean* and/or *whole* foods, as close to the state that God created them as possible. More detailed information about superfoods is included in the Wellness Worksheet section of this book.

Everyday Foods: *Foods with Average Value*

The foods in these lists are acceptable choices on a daily basis. They are just not associated with any specific/remarkable nutrition benefits (or detriments) based on their nutritional value or on current research. In other words, they are OK but still need to take a back seat to the superfoods.

Caution Foods: *Foods with Potential Detriments*

Though all foods can fit into an overall healthy eating pattern (remember, no food is evil), the foods in these lists should, at the very least, be eaten very infrequently and with tremendous restraint—even if you have reached a healthy weight. They are generally higher in calories, added sugars, harmful fats, and/or other harmful additives that have been shown to be detrimental to your health if they hold a prominent place in your daily food choices. Also, because many of these foods are trigger foods that tend to promote overconsumption or binging (sweets, high-fat snack foods, etc.), they have the potential to sabotage your weight-loss and healthy lifestyle efforts in a major way. So it is generally best to avoid these completely if you are trying to lose weight, especially in the initial weeks of following the FP4H plan. Remember, as Christians, we are truly free in Christ to make choices, but boundaries are often necessary to please and honor Him with our bodies, which belong to Him. One of my favorite verses about this topic is 1 Corinthians 6:12. Here it is from the *Amplified Bible*:

> *Everything is permissible for me, but not all things are beneficial. Everything is permissible for me, but I will not be enslaved by anything [and brought under its power, allowing it to control me].*

I will confess to you that there are times when I have allowed certain foods to enslave and control me, and in all the years I have led FP4H groups, I have heard many other people admit to this as well. Satan uses whatever tools seem to work to keep us from putting Christ first in priority. *Anything* that plays this role in our lives has become an idol and must be torn down. So avoid the "caution" foods and show the devil that no *food* is the boss of you—*Jesus* is!

MYplace O FOR NUTRITION

CALORIE INFORMATION FOR ALL FOOD GROUPS

The calorie information provided with each food group list will help you in achieving your First Place for Health meal plan goals. Foods are listed alphabetically in each of the three sections for each group.

The calorie information was obtained from websites endorsed by the United States Department of Agriculture and other reputable public sources of free nutrition information. The data is based on information available at the time this publication was being written and can/will change as manufacturers update product information and submit it to the public agencies. Therefore, what you see on your food package label may differ from what is on these lists. Also, though comprehensive to some degree, the lists cannot possibly contain all of the foods that every FP4H member consumes regularly. For both of these situations, there is space at the end of each food group section to write in your own favorites (using the information on the nutrition facts panel on the food product, restaurant website, etc.). For instance, you may like a whole-grain cereal or bread that isn't listed. Please don't avoid that cereal/bread just because it isn't on this list. There are many healthy options out there and you should feel free to choose foods that are available in your area and that satisfy your taste buds.

Included at the beginning of each food group are average calories for a specified serving from that group. This information is provided to help you with counting foods that may not be listed. For example, if you know that a one-ounce serving of grain is planned to provide an average of 80 calories, and you found a whole-grain bread that you like that is 120 calories for a one-ounce slice, then you would know to count that as 1 ½ ounces of bread, rather than just one ounce. Following the calorie information is a brief description of the group, as well as some nutrition/calorie-control tips for that group.

SECTION 1 THE LIVE-IT FOOD PLAN

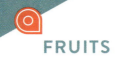

FRUITS

AVERAGE CALORIES (½ CUP) = 50

Write your total daily cups here: _____

Example: For both 1,300-1,400 and 1,700-1,800 calorie levels, this would be 1.5-2 cups.

In general, ½ cup of fruit, ½ cup 100% fruit juice, or ¼ cup dried fruit can be considered as a ½ cup serving from the fruit group.

A large number of studies have shown that eating a diet rich in fruits (and vegetables) as part of an overall healthy diet may reduce the risk for heart disease (including heart attack and stroke) as well as protect against certain types of cancer. Diets rich in foods containing fiber, such as some vegetables and fruits, may also reduce the risk of obesity and type 2 diabetes. Due to these qualities and their overall nutrient density, *all* fruits are superfoods—so there will be no separate list for this food group. A few fruits have been noted (in bold italic print) as being associated with *exceptional* benefits in recent nutrition research, however, so you might want to be sure to try them out!

Nutrition & Calorie Control Tips

- Make most of your choices whole or cut-up fruit rather than juice for the benefits dietary fiber provides and to help ward off hunger. *Eating* your calories tends to keep you feeling fuller and more satisfied than drinking them. Select fruits with more potassium often, such as bananas, plums/prunes, peaches/apricots, and oranges. Consuming foods rich in potassium has been associated with lower blood pressure, reduces the risk of developing kidney stones, and helps to decrease bone loss.

- When choosing canned fruits, select fruit canned in 100% fruit juice or water rather than syrup. (Note: If what you have is packed in syrup, drain it off and rinse before eating; this will eliminate most of the unwanted empty calories.)

SECTION 1   THE LIVE-IT FOOD PLAN

- Vary your fruit choices. Fruits differ in nutrient content. For instance, dried fruits may have more iron, fiber or other nutrients but also tend to have more calories per serving and less vitamin C than many fresh fruits; so, as healthy as they are, you wouldn't want to *only* eat dried fruit.

- Let fruit become your new dessert—you will be surprised how wonderful and sweet it tastes when you start eliminating desserts packed with refined sugars!

FRUIT	QUANTITY	TRACKER VALUE	CALORIES
Apple Slices, Dehydrated	¼ cup	½ cup fruit	86
Apple, Large	1 (about 8 oz)	2 cups fruit	110
Apple, Medium	1 (about 5-6 oz)	1 ¼ cup fruit	72
Apple, Small	1 (less than 4 oz)	1 cup fruit	55
Applesauce, Sweetened	½ cup	½ cup fruit	87
Applesauce, Unsweetened	½ cup	½ cup fruit	51
Apricots, Canned, Lite Syrup	6 halves	½ cup fruit	90
Apricots, Dried	¼ cup	½ cup fruit	78
Apricots, Fresh	2 medium	½ cup fruit	34
Banana Chips	¼ cup	½ cup fruit	66
Banana, Large	8-inch (about 5 oz)	1 cup fruit	121
Banana, Medium	7-inch (about 4 oz)	¾ cup fruit	105
Banana, Small	6 inch (about 3 oz)	½ cup fruit	72
Blackberries	½ cup	½ cup fruit	31
Blueberries	½ cup	½ cup fruit	41
Blueberries, Dried	¼ cup	½ cup fruit	100
Boysenberries	½ cup	½ cup fruit	31
Cantaloupe	½ cup cubes	½ cup fruit	30
Cherries, Dried	¼ cup	½ cup fruit	100
Cherries, Fresh	½ cup	½ cup fruit	37
Cranberries, Dried	¼ cup	½ cup fruit	104
Fruit Cocktail, Canned in Juice	½ cup	½ cup fruit	55

MYplace O FOR NUTRITION

FRUIT	QUANTITY	TRACKER VALUE	CALORIES
Fruit Cocktail, Canned, Lite Syrup	½ cup	½ cup fruit	64
Grapefruit	½ medium	½ cup fruit	41
Grapes, Seedless	½ cup (about 16)	½ cup fruit	52
Honeydew Melon	½ cup cubes	½ cup fruit	32
Juice, Apple	½ cup	½ cup fruit	56
Juice, Grape	½ cup	½ cup fruit	77
Juice, Grapefruit	½ cup	½ cup fruit	47
Juice, Orange	½ cup	½ cup fruit	53
Juice, Pineapple	½ cup	½ cup fruit	70
Juice, Prune	½ cup	½ cup fruit	90
Mango	½ cup cubes	½ cup fruit	54
Nectarine	½ cup slices	½ cup fruit	30
Orange, Fresh, Small	1 (2-inch)	½ cup fruit	42
Orange, Fresh, Medium	1 (2.5-inch)	¾ cup fruit	62
Orange, Fresh, Large	1 (3-inch)	1 cup fruit	86
Oranges, Canned (Mandarin)	½ cup	½ cup fruit	77
Papaya	½ cup cubes	½ cup fruit	27
Peach, Fresh	1 medium	½ cup fruit	38
Peaches, Canned in Juice	½ cup	½ cup fruit	55
Pear, Fresh	1 medium	1 cup fruit	96
Pears, Canned, in juice	½ cup	½ cup fruit	64
Pineapple, Canned in Juice	½ cup	½ cup fruit	60
Pineapple, Fresh	½ cup	½ cup fruit	37
Plum	1 large	½ cup fruit	30
Pomegranate, Raw	½ medium	½ cup fruit	52
Prunes	¼ cup	½ cup fruit	102
Raisins	¼ cup	½ cup fruit	108
Raspberries	½ cup	½ cup fruit	32
Star Fruit (Carambola)	½ cup slices	½ cup fruit	17
Strawberries, Fresh	½ cup	½ cup fruit	23
Strawberries, Frozen, Unsweetened	½ cup, thawed	½ cup fruit	39

SECTION 1 THE LIVE-IT FOOD PLAN

Tangerines/Clementines	1 medium	½ cup fruit	37
Watermelon, Cubes	½ cup cubes	½ cup fruit	23

CAUTION FRUITS

Apple Pie (or other baked fruit pie)	⅛ of 9" pie	½ cup fruit + 2 oz grain + 3 tsp fat	356
Fried Pie, Cherry (or other fried pie)	1 pie	¼ cup fruit + 1 oz grain + 3 tsp fat	272
Peach Cobbler (or other fruit cobbler)	1 cup	1 cup fruit + 2 oz grain + 3 tsp fat	432

PERSONAL FAVORITE FRUITS:

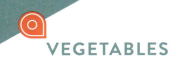

VEGETABLES

AVERAGE CALORIES (FOR ½ CUP): NON-STARCHY = 20 STARCHY = 80

Write your total daily cups here: _____

Example: For 1,300-1,400 calorie level, this would be 1.5-2 cups; 1,700-1,800 would be 2.5-3 cups.

In general, ½ cup of raw or cooked vegetables/vegetable juice or 1 cup of raw leafy greens counts as a ½ cup serving from the vegetable group.

A large number of studies have shown that eating a diet rich in vegetables (and fruits) as part of an overall healthy diet may reduce the risk for heart disease (including heart attack and stroke) as well as protect against certain types of cancer. Diets rich in foods containing fiber, such as some vegetables and fruits, may also reduce the risk of obesity and type 2 diabetes. Due to these qualities and their overall nutrient density, *all* vegetables are superfoods—so there will be no separate list for this food group. A few vegetables have been noted (in bold italic print) as being associated with *exceptional* benefits in recent nutrition research.

Nutrition & Calorie-Control Notes

Most vegetables are naturally low in fat and calories, especially the *non-starchy* ones. Therefore, if you are still hungry after consuming your allowed servings of all the food groups on the FP4H food plan, just eat a few more non-starchy vegetables. As you can see in the chart below, many of them only have 15-30 calories in a ½ cup serving and pack a big nutrition punch, so this is definitely a guilt-free way to ward off the munchies. Because there is a wide variance between the calories in starchy versus non-starchy vegetables, it is wise to limit your intake of starchy vegetables to an average of ½ cup per day (maximum 3 ½ cups per week) to stay within the daily calorie allowance, especially on the 1,300-1,400 and 1,500-1,600 calories levels. Don't panic if you are a starchy-vegetable lover! Because this is an average, it will allow you to choose to eat a medium baked potato (which counts as 1 cup starchy vegetables) one day during the week as long as you avoid starchy vegetables on another day that same week. Also, if you really love beans, remember that if you count your dry beans as protein instead of vegetables (1/4 cup beans = 1 oz. -eq. protein), then you do not need to consider them in the 3 ½ cup weekly maximum of starchy vegetables—the calories are already covered in the protein serving. Don't count them in both groups!

- On the flip side, do *not* avoid certain starchy vegetables just because of the calories. A sweet potato is one of the higher-calorie starchy vegetables, but it is rich in vitamin A and fiber compared to many other vegetables, and...

- Research shows that most people should eat at least 3 cups per week of dark green vegetables and 2 cups per week of red/orange vegetables, so go for the color!

- Focus primarily on fresh, frozen and canned vegetables with no added salt for maximum health benefits and lower sodium intake. People generally eat much more sodium than they need. Be especially careful with this additive if you have high blood pressure, fluid retention issues, and/or a strong family history of heart/kidney disease. Canned vegetables with added salt may be used if absolutely necessary, but consider draining off the liquid and replacing with plain water to reduce sodium content.

- Avoid breaded/battered/fried vegetables as much as possible. You don't need the extra empty calories!

MYplace **O** FOR NUTRITION

VEGETABLES	QUANTITY	TRACKER VALUE	CALORIES
Asparagus	½ cup	½ cup vegetable	20
Artichoke	½ cup	½ cup vegetable	42
Bean Sprouts	½ cup	½ cup vegetable	29
Beans, Green	½ cup	½ cup vegetable	14
Beans, Italian	½ cup	½ cup vegetable	14
Beans, Wax	½ cup	½ cup vegetable	14
Beets	½ cup	½ cup vegetable	37
Broccoli, Cooked	½ cup	½ cup vegetable	17
Broccoli, Fresh	½ cup	½ cup vegetable	12
Cabbage, Cooked	½ cup	½ cup vegetable	17
Cabbage, Raw	½ cup	½ cup vegetable	14
Carrot Juice	½ cup	½ cup vegetable	47
Carrots, Cooked	½ cup	½ cup vegetable	27
Carrots, Fresh	½ cup (1 medium carrot or 6 baby)	½ cup vegetable	25
Cauliflower, Cooked	½ cup	½ cup vegetable	17
Cauliflower, Raw	½ cup	½ cup vegetable	13
Celery, Raw	½ cup	½ cup vegetable	8
Cucumbers	½ cup	½ cup vegetable	7
Eggplant	½ cup	½ cup vegetable	35
Greens, Variety, Cooked	½ cup	½ cup vegetable	18
Mushrooms, Cooked	½ cup	½ cup vegetable	22
Mushrooms, Raw	½ cup	½ cup vegetable	8
Kale, Cooked	½ cup	½ cup vegetable	23

SECTION 1 THE LIVE-IT FOOD PLAN

Okra, Boiled/Steamed (no breading)	½ cup	½ cup vegetable	18
Onions, Green, Chopped	½ cup	½ cup vegetable	16
Onions, White or Yellow, Raw, Chopped	½ cup	½ cup vegetable	34
Onions, White or Yellow, Cooked	½ cup	½ cup vegetable	46
Peas and Carrots	½ cup	½ cup vegetable	38
Peppers, Bell, Raw	½ cup	½ cup vegetable	9
Pumpkin	½ cup	½ cup vegetable	42
Sauerkraut	½ cup	½ cup vegetable	14
Snow Peas	½ cup	½ cup vegetable	34
Spaghetti Sauce (1st ingred. Tomatoes)	½ cup	½ cup vegetable	51
Spinach, Cooked	½ cup	½ cup vegetable	30
Squash, Spaghetti	½ cup	½ cup vegetable	19
Squash, Yellow/Summer, Boiled/Grilled	½ cup	½ cup vegetable	18
Squash, Zucchini	½ cup	½ cup vegetable	18
Tomato Juice	½ cup	½ cup vegetable	11
Tomatoes, Cooked	½ cup	½ cup vegetable	22
Tomatoes, Fresh	½ cup (1 small, or 6 cherry, or 10 grape)	½ cup vegetable	16
Turnips, Cooked	½ cup	½ cup vegetable	17
Vegetable Juice (Ex: V-8)	½ cup	½ cup vegetable	22
Vegetable Soup w/Beef, Canned	1 cup (water added)	½ cup vegetable	78

VEGETABLES - RAW / LEAFY

Kale, Chopped	1 cup	½ cup vegetable	33
Lettuce, Escarole	1 cup	½ cup vegetable	8
Lettuce, Endive	1 cup	½ cup vegetable	6

MYplace O FOR NUTRITION

VEGETABLES - RAW / LEAFY			
Lettuce, Iceberg	1 cup	½ cup vegetable	8
Lettuce, Romaine	1 cup	½ cup vegetable	7
Spinach	1 cup	½ cup vegetable	7

VEGETABLES - STARCHY			
Avocado, chopped	½ cup	½ cup vegetable + 2 tsp. oil	120
Beans, Black	½ cup	½ cup vegetable	111
Beans, Great Northern	½ cup	½ cup vegetable	121
Beans, Kidney	½ cup	½ cup vegetable	108
Beans, Lima, Green/Baby	½ cup	½ cup vegetable	104
Beans, Navy	½ cup	½ cup vegetable	121
Beans, Pinto	½ cup	½ cup vegetable	123
Beans, Refried, Fat Free	½ cup	½ cup vegetable	100
Chickpeas	½ cup	½ cup vegetable	148
Corn, Cream Style	½ cup	½ cup vegetable	92
Corn, Whole Kernel	½ cup	½ cup vegetable	88
Hominy	½ cup	½ cup vegetable	70
Hummus	¼ cup	¼ cup vegetable + 1 tsp oil	109
Lentils	½ cup	½ cup vegetable	110
Olives, Black	¼ cup	¼ cup vegetable + 1 tsp oil	35
Olives, Green	¼ cup	¼ cup vegetable + 1 tsp oil	48

SECTION 1 THE LIVE-IT FOOD PLAN

Peas, Black-eyed	½ cup	½ cup vegetable	79
Peas, English/Green	½ cup	½ cup vegetable	66
Peas, Purple Hull	½ cup	½ cup vegetable	79
Plantain	½ cup	½ cup vegetable	137
Pork and Beans	½ cup	¼ cup vegetable	124
Potatoes, White, Strips/Fries, Frozen, Baked	8-10 medium strips	½ cup vegetable + 1 tsp oil	140
Potatoes, White, Baked or Boiled	1 med.(8oz)	1 cup vegetable	121
Potatoes, White, Mashed (no marg.)	½ cup	½ cup vegetable	97
Soybeans (Edamame)	½ cup	½ cup vegetable	95
Squash, Acorn	½ cup	½ cup vegetable	40
Squash, Butternut	½ cup	½ cup vegetable	40
Sweet Potatoes/Yams, Mashed	½ cup	½ cup vegetable	80
Sweet Potato, Baked	1 large	1 cup vegetable	162
Vegetable Soup, Canned	1 cup	½ cup vegetable	82

CAUTION VEGETABLES

Beans, Refried, Regular (with lard)	½ cup	½ cup vegetable + 2 tsp fat	182
Okra, Fried (breaded)	½ cup	¼ cup vegetable + ½ oz grain + 1 tsp oil	87
Potato Chips, Baked	1 small bag (1oz)	½ cup vegetable + 1 tsp oil	130
Potato Chips, Fried	1 small bag (1oz)	½ cup vegetable + 2 tsp oil	150
Potatoes, French Fries, Fried	1 cup or 1 small order	½ cup vegetable + 2 tsp oil	265
Squash, Yellow, Breaded & Fried	½ cup	½ cup vegetable + 1 oz grain + 3 tsp oil	194

MYplace ○ FOR NUTRITION

PERSONAL FAVORITE VEGETABLES:

SECTION 1 THE LIVE-IT FOOD PLAN

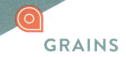

GRAINS

Average Calories (1 oz) Grain = 80

Write your total daily ounces here: _____

(Example: For 1,300-1,400 calorie level, this would be 5 oz; for 1,700-1,800, this would be 6-7 oz.)

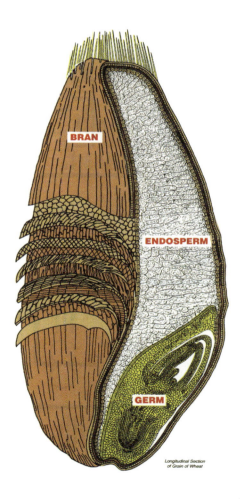

Longitudinal Section of Grain of Wheat

Any food made from wheat, rice, oats, cornmeal, or another cereal grain is a grain product. Grains may be divided into two subgroups—whole grains and refined grains. *Whole* grains contain the entire grain kernel—the bran, germ, and endosperm (see diagram). People who eat whole grains as part of a healthy diet have a reduced risk of many chronic diseases. *Refined* grains have been milled, a process that removes the bran and germ. This is done to give grains a finer texture and to improve their shelf life, but it also removes dietary fiber, iron, and many B vitamins. On the First Place for Health Live It food plan, at least *half* of all the grains you eat should be whole grains, and preferably more!

SECTION 1 THE LIVE-IT FOOD PLAN

Nutrition & Calorie-Control Tips

○ The easiest way to determine if something qualifies as a whole grain is to check the ingredient listing. If a whole grain (such as whole-wheat flour, whole corn, whole oats, or brown rice) is listed *first*, it qualifies. In the list below, only whole grains are listed in the superfoods section.

○ Watch for added fats/oils in grain products. These are especially common in crackers, snack foods, and quick breads. If a grain product has 5 grams of fat in a one ounce serving, then you will need to also count that food as one teaspoon of healthy oil or other fat. Some foods in the list below (example: Wheat Thins/Ritz crackers, Grands Biscuits) fall into this category. This is the reason that *many* times you don't have any "healthy oil" servings left to eat individually during a day—because they are all already used up in the grain foods you consume!

○ If you usually follow a gluten-free eating plan (for Celiac disease or for gluten sensitivity/gastrointestinal symptoms), feel free to choose gluten-free products for your grains. Just be sure to stay with a one-ounce dry portion size for each grain serving (or half cup of a cooked cereal grain), and try to stay with whole gluten-free grains (like brown rice, quinoa, or whole-oat products that are certified as gluten-free) as much as possible.

GRAINS	QUANTITY	TRACKER VALUE	CALORIES
SUPERFOOD GRAINS			
Bagel, Whole Wheat	1 small	2 ½ oz grain	173
Barley, Cooked, Hulled/Hull-less	½ cup	1 oz grain	108
Bread, Gluten Free (whole grain 1st ingredient)	1 slice	1 oz grain	75
Bread, Multigrain (whole grain 1st ingredient)	1 reg. slice	1 oz grain	65
Bread, Whole Wheat, Diet	1 slice	½ oz grain	50
Bread, Whole Wheat, Regular	1 reg. slice	1 oz grain	69

MYplace ○ FOR NUTRITION

GRAINS - SUPERFOODS	QUANTITY	TRACKER VALUE	CALORIES
Bulgur, Cooked (cracked wheat)	½ cup	1 oz grain	56
Bun, Hamburger, Whole Wheat	1 bun	1 ½ oz grain	96
Bun, Hot Dog, Whole Wheat	1 bun	1 ½ oz grain	96
Cereal, All Bran	½ cup	1 oz grain	78
Cereal, Bran Flakes	1 cup	1 oz grain	144
Cereal, Cheerios	1 cup	1 oz grain	111
Cereal, Corn Flakes	1 cup	1 oz grain	90
Cereal, Corn or Wheat Chex	1 cup	1 oz grain	143
Cereal, Grape Nuts	¼ cup	1 oz grain	98
Cereal, Kashi, Puffed	1 cup	1 oz grain	88
Cereal, Puffed Wheat	1 cup	½ oz grain	44
Cereal, Raisin Bran	1 cup	1 oz grain	195
Cereal, Rice Chex	1 cup	1 oz grain	124
Cereal, Rice Krispies	1 cup	1 oz grain	94
Cereal, Shredded Wheat	½ cup	1 oz grain	85
Chips, Tortilla, Baked	8 chips	1 oz grain	87
Chips, Tortilla, Regular	7 each	1 oz grain + 1.5 tsp oil	160
Crackers, Gluten Free, Crunchmaster	16 each	1 oz grain + 1 tsp oil	130
Crackers, Triscuits, Regular	6 crackers	1 oz grain + 1 tsp oil	120
Crackers, Triscuits, Reduced Fat	7 crackers	1 oz grain + 1 tsp oil	120
Crackers, Wheat Thins, Regular	14 crackers	1 oz grain + 1 tsp oil	140
Crackers, Wheat Thins, Reduced Fat	14 crackers	1 oz grain + 1 tsp oil	130
English Muffin, Whole Wheat	½ medium	1 oz grain	65
Graham Crackers	4 squares	1 oz grain	118

SECTION 1 THE LIVE-IT FOOD PLAN

Granola Bar, Regular (whole grain 1st ingredient)	1 bar	½ oz grain + 1 tsp oil	130
Granola Bar, Low Fat (whole grain 1st ingredient)	1 bar	½ oz grain + ½ tsp oil	95
Granola, Low Fat	½ cup	1 oz grain + 2 tsp oil	209
Millet, Cooked	½ cup	1 oz grain	103
Oatmeal, Flavored, Cooked with Water	½ cup	1 oz grain	106
Oatmeal, Plain, Cooked with Water	½ cup	1 oz grain	73
Pancakes, Whole Wheat	1 (5-inch)	1 oz grain	91
Pasta, Whole Wheat	½ cup cooked	1 oz grain	86
Popcorn, Fat Free or Air Popped	3 cups	1 oz grain	93
Popcorn, Lite, Microwave	3 cups	1 oz grain + ½ tsp oil	110
Quinoa, Cooked	½ cup	1 oz grain	111
Rice, Brown, Cooked	½ cup	1 oz grain	107
Rice, Wild	½ cup	1 oz grain	65
Roll, Whole Wheat	1 small	1 oz grain	82
Taco Shells (whole corn 1st ingredient)	2 shells	1 oz grain + 1 tsp oil	124
Tortillas, Corn	1 (6-inch)	1 oz grain	53
Tortillas, Whole Wheat	1 (6-inch)	1 oz grain	70
Waffles, Bran/Multi-Grain/Wheat	1 (4-inch)	1 oz grain	115
EVERYDAY GRAINS			
Animal Crackers, Plain (unfrosted)	1 oz	1 oz grain	127
Bagel, Cinnamon Raisin	1 small	2 ½ oz grain	189
Bagel, White, Plain	1 small	2 ½ oz grain	181

MYplace ○ FOR NUTRITION

GRAINS - EVERYDAY	QUANTITY	TRACKER VALUE	CALORIES
Barley, Cooked, Pearled	½ cup	1 oz grain	99
Biscuit, Canned	1 small	½ oz grain	66
Biscuit, Canned	1 medium	1 oz grain + ½ tsp fat	100
Bread, French	1 reg. slice	1 oz grain	59
Bread, Gluten Free (tapioca/potato flour/white rice 1st ingredient)	1 slice	1 oz grain	70
Bread, Rye	1 reg. slice	1 oz grain	67
Bread, White, Diet	1 thin slice	½ oz grain	48
Bread, White, Regular	1 reg. slice	1 oz grain	69
Bun, Hamburger, White	1 medium	1 ½ oz grain	120
Bun, Hot Dog, White	1 medium	1 ½ oz grain	120
Cereal, Variety, Sweetened, Non-whole Grain	1 cup	1 oz grain	150
Cornbread	1 medium muffin or 2" square	1 ½ oz grain + 1 tsp oil	174
Crackers, Cheese Flavored	½ cup	1 oz grain + 1 tsp oil	133
Crackers, Cheese Flavored, Red. Fat	½ cup	1 oz grain + ½ tsp oil	100
Crackers, Gluten-free (tapioca/ potato flour/white rice 1st ingredient)	8 crackers	1 oz grain + 1 tsp oil	140
Crackers, Ritz, Regular	7 rounds	1 oz grain + 1 tsp oil	112
Crackers, Ritz, Reduced Fat	7 rounds	1 oz grain + ½ tsp oil	71
Crackers, Saltines	6 crackers	1 oz grain	78
Cream of Wheat, Cooked	½ cup	1 oz grain	55
English Muffin, White	½ medium	1 oz grain	68
Grits, Hominy, Cooked	½ cup	1 oz grain	56

Pancakes, White	1 (5-inch)	1 oz grain	91
Pasta, Regular (noodles, macaroni)	½ cup cooked	1 oz grain	98
Pretzels, Hard	½ cup	1 oz grain	76
Pretzels, Soft	1 medium	4 oz grain	194
Raisin Bread	1 reg. slice	1 oz grain	71
Rice, White, Cooked	½ cup	1 oz grain	102
Roll, White	1 small	1 oz grain	78
Soup, Chicken Noodle (water added)	1 cup	½ oz grain	75
Tortillas, White Flour	1 (6-inch)	1 oz grain	110
Waffles, Frozen, Regular	1 (4-inch)	1 oz grain	103

CAUTION GRAINS

Biscuit Canned, Large Size	1 large (ex: Pillsbury Grands)	2 oz grain + 1 tsp fat	180
Biscuit, Restaurant/Fast Food	1 regular	1 ½ oz grain + 1 ½ tsp fat	180
Cake, no Frosting	1/12 sheet cake	1 oz grain + 2 tsp fat	150
Cake, with Frosting	1/12 sheet cake	1 oz grain + 4 tsp fat	400
Croissant	1 medium	2 oz grain + 2 tsp fat	251
Doughnut, Cake-type, Frosted	1 medium	1 oz grain + 4 tsp fat	251
Doughnut, Cake-type, Unfrosted	1 medium	1 oz grain + 3 tsp fat	198
Doughnut, Raised, Frosted	1 medium	1 oz grain + 4 tsp fat	275
Doughnut, Raised, Jelly-filled	1 medium	1 oz grain + 3 tsp fat	221
Muffin, Blueberry or Banana, Purchased	1 medium	2 oz grain + 3 tsp fat	295
Popcorn, Butter/Theater Style	3 cups	1 oz grain + 2 tsp fat	219

MYplace O FOR NUTRITION

PERSONAL FAVORITE GRAINS:

SECTION 1 THE LIVE-IT FOOD PLAN

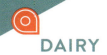
DAIRY

Average Calories (1 cup) = 90

Write your total daily cups here: _____

(Example: For the 1,300-1,400 calorie level, this would be 2-3 cups; for 1,700-1,800, this would be 3 cups.)

All fluid milk products and many foods made from milk are considered part of this food group. In general, 1 cup of milk, yogurt or soy milk, 1 ½ ounces of natural cheese, or 2 ounces of processed cheese can be considered as a 1 cup serving from the dairy group. These foods provide many health benefits—especially improved bone health and reduced risk of osteoporosis because of their high calcium content. Consistent, daily intake of dairy products is also associated with a reduced risk of cardiovascular disease and type 2 diabetes, and with lower blood pressure in adults.

Nutrition & Calorie-Control Tips

- It is expected that you will choose *fat-free* products for *at least half* of your dairy total for the day, to stay within the calorie estimates; these choices also help eliminate unhealthy saturated fats from your diet. To keep calories in line, you may have to trade off the items that are most important to you. For instance, if you can handle fat-free (skim) milk and fat-free yogurt but just can't tolerate fat-free cheese, just choose the 2% cheese as one of your higher-calorie dairy choices.

- For the purposes of the food plan, a one-cup serving from the milk group is expected to provide you with 30% of the recommended daily intake of calcium. Check your milk product's label for specifics. If it provides 20%, then it would count as 2/3 cup milk, 15% would count as ½ cup milk, and so forth.

SECTION 1 THE LIVE-IT FOOD PLAN

○ If you are unable to drink cow's milk due to milk allergy or lactose intolerance (or if you follow a vegan style of eating), you may substitute soy or almond milk products, also shown in the list below. In order to make sure that you are getting the equivalent calcium, however, check the nutrition label. The substitute needs to provide at least 30% of the recommend daily value of calcium in a one cup serving to be equal in that nutrient. If your substitution does not have 8 grams of protein in a one cup serving (like cow's milk), you may also need to add an additional ounce of cooked protein during the day to meet your protein needs.

DAIRY	QUANTITY	TRACKER VALUE	CALORIES
SUPERFOODS			
Milk, Nonfat, Dry	⅓ cup powder	1 cup milk	92
Milk, Evaporated, Fat Free/Skim	½ cup	1 cup milk	100
Milk, Fat Free/Skim	1 cup	1 cup milk	83
Yogurt, Fat Free, Greek, No Sugar Added	5-6 oz container	½ cup milk	80
Yogurt, Fat Free, Greek, No Sugar Added	1 cup	⅔ cup milk	130
Yogurt, Fat Free, No Sugar Added	6 oz container	⅔ cup milk	80
Yogurt, Fat Free, No Sugar Added	1 cup	1 cup milk	98
EVERYDAY DAIRY FOODS			
Almond Milk, Calcium Fortified (30%)	1 cup	1 cup milk	56
Buttermilk, Cultured, Fat Free	1 cup	1 cup milk	98
Cheese Spread, Velveeta, 2%	1 oz	½ cup milk	49
Cheese, American, 2%	1 slice (¾ oz)	½ cup milk	50
Cheese, American, Fat Free	1 slice (¾ oz)	½ cup milk	30
Cheese, Cheddar, 2%	1 oz	⅔ cup milk	80
Cheese, Cheddar, Fat Free	1 oz	⅔ cup milk	42

MYplace O FOR NUTRITION

DAIRY - EVERYDAY	QUANTITY	TRACKER VALUE	CALORIES
Cheese, Cottage, Low Fat/1%	½ cup	¼ cup milk	81
Cheese, Cream, Fat Free	2 oz	¾ cup milk	52
Cheese, Feta/Goat	¼ cup	¾ cup milk	99
Cheese, Mozzarella, Part Skim	1 oz	⅔ cup milk	86
Cheese, Parmesan, Grated	2 Tbsp.	¼ cup milk	43
Cheese, Swiss, 2%	1 oz	⅔ cup milk	51
Hot Cocoa Mix, Sugar Free, with Water	1 packet	¼ cup milk	57
Milk, Low Fat (1%)	1 cup	1 cup milk	102
Pudding, Sugar Free (fat-free milk)	½ cup	½ cup milk	81
Pudding, Sweetened (fat-free milk)	½ cup	½ cup milk	105
Sour Cream, Fat Free	1 cup	¾ cup milk	168
Soy Milk, Plain, Calcium Fortified (30%)	1 cup	1 cup milk	108
Yogurt, Frozen, Nonfat, No Sugar Added	1 cup	¾ cup milk	199

CAUTION DAIRY FOODS

	QUANTITY	TRACKER VALUE	CALORIES
Cheese Spread, Velveeta, Regular	1 oz	½ cup milk + 1 tsp fat	82
Cheese, American, Regular	1 slice (¾ oz)	⅓ cup milk + 1 tsp fat	70
Cheese, Cheddar, Regular	1 oz	⅔ cup milk + 1.5 tsp fat	114
Cheese, Cottage, Regular/4%	½ cup	¼ cup milk + 1.5 tsp fat	108
Cheese, Ricotta, Regular	¼ cup	½ cup milk + 1 tsp fat	96
Cheese, Swiss, Regular	1 oz	⅔ cup milk + 1.5 tsp fat	113
Ice Cream, Lite/Reduced Fat	1 cup	¾ cup milk + 2 tsp fat	216
Ice Cream, Regular	1 cup	¼ cup milk + 2 tsp fat	267

SECTION 1 THE LIVE-IT FOOD PLAN

Milk, Evaporated, Whole	½ cup	1 cup milk + 2 tsp fat	160
Milk, Reduced Fat (2%)	1 cup	1 cup milk + 1 tsp fat	122
Milk, Whole	1 cup	1 cup milk + 2 tsp fat	140
Yogurt, Frozen, Low Fat (sugar-sweetened)	1 cup	¾ cup milk + 1 tsp fat	214
Yogurt, Plain, Regular	1 cup	1 cup milk + 1 tsp fat	138

PERSONAL FAVORITE DAIRY:

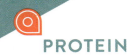

PROTEIN

Average Calories (1 oz) = 70

Write in your total daily ounces here: _____

(Example: For the 1,300-1,400 calorie level, this would be 4 oz; for the 1,700-1,800 level, this would be 5-5.5 oz.)

All foods made from meat, poultry, seafood, beans and peas, eggs, processed soy products, nuts and seeds are considered part of this group. In general, 1 ounce of cooked meat, poultry or fish, ¼ cup cooked beans, 1 egg, 1 tablespoon nut butter, or ½ oz nuts or seeds counts as a 1 ounce serving. These foods provide protein as well as many minerals and B vitamins necessary for the health and maintenance of your body.

Nutrition & Calorie-Control Tips

- Select a *variety* of protein foods over the course of each week to improve nutrient intake and health benefits.

- Remember, the weights on meat/poultry/fish are *after cooking* (and without any bones), so don't cheat yourself by weighing the raw product! Use an inexpensive food scale to check weights so that you stay within your daily limits.

- Prepare meat/poultry/fish items by removing any visible fat and using low-fat cooking methods, such as grilling, roasting, broiling, and baking. You may also use a nonstick cooking spray to cook them in a skillet on top of the stove.

- The vast majority of your choices from this group need to be very lean or low fat. Choosing foods from this group that are high in saturated fat (see "Caution" foods) may have heart-health implications (besides adding more unnecessary calories!). If you are not sure whether or not certain cuts of beef or pork are lean (due to no notations on the package), look for visible fat con-

SECTION 1 **THE LIVE-IT FOOD PLAN**

tent. The white exterior and marbling (white specks) within the flesh indicate a higher fat content.

○ Try to include at least 8 oz of cooked seafood per week, and choose non-meat sources of protein (such as beans/peas and nuts) often. These protein choices as part of a diet filled with fruits, vegetables, and whole grains is called a Mediterranean style of eating and is associated with a vast number of health benefits (and disease prevention) in many recent studies.

○ Processed meats, such as ham, sausage, hot dogs, and deli meats, have added sodium. Check the nutrition-facts labels to help limit your sodium intake.

○ A diet high in consumption of highly processed meats and other processed foods has been associated with increased chronic inflammation in the body, so read the ingredient labels for the best choices on processed items. Better yet, stay with plain (unprocessed) fresh or frozen meats as much as possible. Items with long ingredient lists that you can't even begin to pronounce usually are *not* the ideal choices for your health. Stay with foods with simple ingredients—closest to their natural state. This advice goes for *all* of the food groups.

○ Choose unsalted varieties of nuts and seeds to keep sodium intake low.

PROTEIN SUPERFOODS	QUANTITY	TRACKER VALUE	CALORIES
Almond Butter	1 Tbsp	1 oz protein + 1 tsp oil	98
Almonds	½ oz (12)	1 oz protein + 1 tsp oil	82
Beans, Black	¼ cup	1 oz protein	55
Beans, Great Northern	¼ cup	1 oz protein	60
Beans, Kidney	¼ cup	1 oz protein	54
Beans, Navy	¼ cup	1 oz protein	60
Beans, Pinto	¼ cup	1 oz protein	61

MYplace **O** FOR NUTRITION

PROTEIN – SUPERFOODS	QUANTITY	TRACKER VALUE	CALORIES
Beans, Refried, Fat Free	¼ cup	1 oz protein	50
Cashews	½ oz (9)	1 oz protein + 1 tsp oil	83
Chia Seeds	1 Tbsp.	1 oz protein + 1 tsp oil	69
Chickpeas	¼ cup	1 oz protein	74
Fish, Baked (unbreaded), Cod/Pollock	1 oz	1 oz protein	41
Fish, Salmon, Baked or Broiled	1 oz	1 oz protein	48
Fish, Salmon, Smoked	1 oz	1 oz protein	33
Hazelnuts/Filberts	½ oz (10)	1 oz protein + 1 tsp oil	88
Hummus	¼ cup	1 ½ oz protein + 1 tsp oil	109
Lentils, Cooked	¼ cup	1 oz protein	55
Mixed Nuts	½ oz (2T)	1 oz protein + 1 tsp oil	102
Peanut Butter	1 Tbsp	1 oz protein + 1 tsp oil	96
Peanuts	½ oz (2T)	1 oz protein + 1 tsp oil	106
Pecans	½ oz (10 halves)	1 oz protein + 1 tsp oil	98
Pistachios	¼ cup (24, in shell)	1 oz protein + 1 tsp oil	82
Seeds, Flax	2 Tbsp	1 ½ oz protein + 1 tsp oil	97
Seeds, Sunflower	½ oz (2T)	1 oz protein + 1 tsp oil	93
Soybeans	¼ cup	1 oz protein	64
Tofu	¼ cup	1 oz protein	38
Tuna, Canned in Oil, Drained	¼ cup	1 ½ oz protein	72
Tuna, Canned in Water	¼ cup	1 ½ oz protein	33
Walnuts	½ oz (7 halves)	1 oz protein + 1 tsp oil	93

SECTION 1 THE LIVE-IT FOOD PLAN

EVERYDAY PROTEIN FOODS

Bacon, Turkey	2 slices	1 oz protein	84
Beef, Lean Steak or Roast	1 oz	1 oz protein	56
Beef, Ground, 85% Lean (round)	1 oz	1 oz protein	65
Beef, Ground, 90% Lean	1 oz	1 oz protein	57
Beef, Ground, 95% Lean	1 oz	1 oz protein	46
Beef, Roast, Deli Sliced	1 oz	1 oz protein	50
Canadian Bacon	1 oz	1 oz protein	43
Chicken, Dark Protein, No Skin	1 oz	1 oz protein	66
Chicken, White Protein, No Skin	1 oz	1 oz protein	55
Chili, Canned, Turkey w/Beans	1 cup	3 oz protein + $\frac{3}{4}$ c vegetable	210
Egg Whites	2 whites	1 oz protein	34
Egg, Whole, Boiled/Poached (no fat)	1 whole	1 oz protein	78
Egg, Whole, Pan-Fried/Scrambled with Nonstick Cooking Spray	1 whole	1 oz protein	80
Fish, Baked (unbreaded), Catfish	1 oz	1 oz protein	46
Ham, Pork, Deli, Extra Lean	1 oz	1 oz protein	37
Ham, Pork, Deli, Regular	1 oz	1 oz protein	45
Ham, Pork, Smoked	1 oz	1 oz protein	45
Hot Dog Wiener, Low Fat (turkey, beef)	1 wiener	2 oz protein	130
Lobster	1 oz	1 oz protein	28
Pork Loin, Baked/Broiled/Grilled	1 oz	1 oz protein	59

MYp ace ○ FOR NUTRITION

PROTEIN - EVERYDAY	QUANTITY	TRACKER VALUE	CALORIES
Sausage, Turkey, Link	¼ cup slices	1 oz protein	59
Scallops, Baked/Broiled/Grilled	1 oz	1 oz protein	37
Shrimp, Broiled/Grilled/Sauteed	1 oz	1 oz protein	43
Shrimp, Steamed/Boiled	1 oz	1 oz protein	39
Turkey or Chicken, Deli Sliced	1 oz	1 oz protein	29
Turkey, Ground	1 oz	1 oz protein	65
Turkey, Roasted, White Protein	1 oz	1 oz protein	44
Turkey, Roasted, White/Dark Mix	1 oz	1 oz protein	47
Vegetable Beef Soup, Canned	1 cup (water added)	½ oz protein + ½ cup veg.	78
CAUTION PROTEIN FOODS			
Bacon, Pork	2 slices	½ oz protein + 1 tsp fat	87
Beef, Ground, 80% Lean (chuck)	1 oz	1 oz protein + ½ tsp fat	69
Beef, Ground, Regular (70-80% lean)	1 oz	1 oz protein + 1 tsp fat	80
Bratwurst, Beef	1 oz	1 oz protein + 1 tsp fat	84
Bratwurst, Pork	1 oz	1 oz protein + 1 tsp fat	94
Chicken, Fried, With Skin	1 oz	1 oz protein + 1 tsp fat	80
Hot Dog Wiener, Regular (pork, beef)	1 wiener	1 ½ oz protein + 1 tsp fat	186
Egg, Whole, Fried with Oil or Fat Added	1 whole	1 oz protein + ½ tsp fat	89
Sausage, Polish, Regular	¼ cup slices	1 oz protein + 1 tsp fat	117
Sausage, Pork, Brown & Serve	1 patty	½ oz protein + 1 tsp fat	107
Shrimp, Fried, Battered	2 oz	1 oz protein + ½ oz grain + 1 tsp oil	167

SECTION 1 THE LIVE-IT FOOD PLAN

PERSONAL FAVORITE PROTEIN:

HEALTHY OILS / OTHER FATS

AVERAGE CALORIES (1 TSP) = 45

Write in your total daily teaspoons here: _____

(Example: For the 1,300-1,400 calorie level, this would be 4 tsp.; for the 1,700-1,800 level, this would be 5 tsp.)

Oils are fats that are liquid at room temperature, like the vegetable oils used in cooking. Oils come from many different plants and from fish. Oils are not really a food group, but they provide essential nutrients and contain monounsaturated and polyunsaturated ("good") fats, so are included in our recommendations for a healthy eating plan.

Solid fats are fats that are solid at room temperature, like beef fat, butter and shortening. Solid fats mainly come from animal foods but can also be made from vegetable oils through a process called hydrogenation. These fats contain more saturated and/or trans fats, which tend to raise LDL ("bad") cholesterol levels in the blood, which in turn increases the risk of heart disease.

Nutrition & Calorie-Control Tips

- Based on the above information, it is highly recommended that the vast majority of your fat choices come from the healthy oils. These are listed in the first two lists below ("Superfoods" and "Everyday Healthy Oils"). However, since people do tend to consume at least *some* extra saturated fats, and these calories need to be counted somewhere in your plan, we have chosen to provide the saturated fat choices in the "Caution Fats" list below.

- USDA recommends that *less than 10%* of your total calories come from saturated fats. To put this in perspective, on a 1,300-1,400 calorie plan, you would need to consume no more than 130-140 calories per day from saturated fats (or about 15 grams of saturated fat). The way the FP4H calorie levels are planned, some of these will be accounted for in your meat and milk

SECTION 1 **THE LIVE-IT FOOD PLAN**

choices, depending on what items you choose from those groups. Therefore, it is *very* easy to exceed recommendations and have no room for extra solid fats, like butter or regular sour cream, unless you consistently choose very lean meats (or non-meat) sources of protein and fat-free dairy products.

○ Your choices from both healthy oils *and* other fats should be counted on your Live It Tracker. Be sure to note where additional teaspoons of oil (healthy fat) or teaspoons of fat (unhealthy fat) are listed with other food group choices when tallying up your daily total for this group.

HEALTHY OILS & OTHER FATS - EVERYDAY	QUANTITY	TRACKER VALUE	CALORIES
SUPERFOODS			
Almonds	1 Tbsp	1 tsp oil	42
Avocado	¼ cup	1 tsp oil + ¼ cup vegetable	60
Cashews	2 Tbsp	1 tsp fat	44
Hazelnuts/Filberts	1 Tbsp	1 tsp oil	50
Mixed Nuts	1 Tbsp	1 tsp oil	44
Oil, Olive (regular or extra virgin)	1 tsp	1 tsp oil	40
Peanut Butter	1 ½ tsp	1 tsp oil	48
Pecans	1 Tbsp	1 tsp oil	48
Peanuts	1 Tbsp	1 tsp oil	43
Sunflower Seeds	1 Tbsp	1 tsp oil	42
Walnuts	1 Tbsp	1 tsp oil	46
EVERYDAY HEALTHY OILS			
Margarine, Stick, Lite, 0 Trans fat	1 Tbsp	1 tsp oil	50
Margarine Spread, Tub, Lite, 0 trans fat	1 Tbsp	1 tsp oil	50
Margarine, Tub, Regular, 0 trans fat	1 tsp	1 tsp oil	34
Mayonnaise, Lite	1 Tbsp	1 tsp oil	36
Mayonnaise, Regular	1 Tbsp	2 tsp oil	99
Oil, Vegetable (Canola, Corn, Soybean)	1 tsp	1 tsp oil	40

MYplace **O** FOR NUTRITION

HEALTHY OILS & OTHER FATS - EVERYDAY	QUANTITY	TRACKER VALUE	CALORIES
Salad Dressing, Blue Cheese	1 Tbsp	2 tsp oil	98
Salad Dressing, Italian, Regular	1 Tbsp	1 tsp oil	43
Salad Dressing, Plain (Miracle Whip)	1 Tbsp	1 tsp oil	57
Salad Dressing, Plain, Lite	2 Tbsp	1 tsp oil	48
Salad Dressing, Ranch, Lite	2 Tbsp	1 tsp oil	48
Salad Dressing, Ranch, Regular	1 Tbsp	1 tsp oil	71
Salad Dressing, Thousand Island, Regular	1 Tbsp	1 tsp oil	58
CAUTION FATS			
Alfredo Sauce, Prepared	2 Tbsp	3 tsp fat	137
Bacon, Cooked	1 medium slice	1 tsp fat	40
Butter	1 Tbsp	2 tsp fat	102
Cream Cheese, Regular	2 Tbsp	1 tsp fat	50
Half & Half	2 Tbsp	1 tsp fat	40
Sour Cream, Lite	2 Tbsp	1 tsp fat	44
Sour Cream, Regular	2 Tbsp	$1\frac{1}{2}$ tsp fat	56

PERSONAL FAVORITE HEALTHY OILS & OTHER FATS

SECTION 1 THE LIVE-IT FOOD PLAN

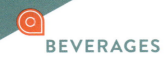

BEVERAGES

AVERAGE CALORIES (1 CUP OR 8 OZ) = 0

There's no doubt about it—the foods you consume every day can have a significant impact on your health, and the same is true of the beverages you choose!

It is important to provide your body with adequate fluids every day for vital physical functions, such as maintaining your internal temperature and blood pressure, cushioning joints and organs, helping with digestion/absorption/transport of nutrients (including the breakdown of fat!), and getting rid of harmful substances (toxins).

How much water do we need?

Generally, women should consume a total of 90 ounces of water per day, or the equivalent of about 11 (8 oz) glasses. Men should consume a total of 123 ounces per day, or about 16 (8 oz) glasses. However, bear in mind that many *foods* have a high water content (especially fruits and vegetables), and foods usually provide about 20% of your water intake, so this will reduce your beverage fluid needs to about 9 cups (8 oz each) for women and 13 cups for men.[1]

So, what should you be drinking to get these 9 or 13 cups? The most current nutrition research shows that the most Super Beverages are:

1. Water
2. Tea (green, black, white)
3. Coffee

What About Caffeine?

Though consumption of a moderate amount of caffeine daily (the amount in 2-3 cups of brewed coffee) has been shown to be safe and even beneficial in some studies, bear in mind that consuming *too much* caffeine may be unwise. It can

SECTION 1 THE LIVE-IT FOOD PLAN

aggravate several health conditions, including gastro-esophageal reflux, migraine headaches, irregular heartbeat, sleep disturbance, and benign fibrocystic breast disease. However, if you are sensitive to caffeine, you can still gain many of the healthy antioxidant benefits from *decaffeinated* coffee and tea. Just remember that "having a little coffee with your creamer and sugar" will offset its potential health benefits, so skip the additions or keep them to a minimum. See the "Extras & Additions" section for the calorie contribution of many of these items.

Recording Fluids on Your Live It Tracker

Because of the importance of getting enough water and other healthy fluids to stay hydrated, we are going to ask you to record your daily cups of these beverages on your Live It Tracker. You may count water, tea, and coffee, but nothing else. You may record regular (caffeinated) coffee and tea *up to 3 cups per day* to meet your daily goal, but the remaining fluids recorded should only be water and decaffeinated tea/coffee.

Avoid Sugar-Sweetened Beverages!

Many experts believe that sugar-sweetened beverages—soda, sweet teas and coffees, energy drinks, sports drinks, and fruit-flavored beverages—may be a major contributing factor to the our nation's obesity problem, as well as to the growing numbers of people suffering from type 2 diabetes. The most current USDA Dietary Guidelines recommend that added sugars be limited to 10% of your daily calories; so for a 1,300-1,400 meal plan, this would be 130-140 calories, or about 8 teaspoons (32 grams). Many of these added sugars will actually be present in many grain items and other processed foods that you may not realize they are in—even products like canned soups and spaghetti sauce—so there really just isn't any room for sugar-sweetened beverages! Did you know that if you consume an extra 150-calorie beverage twice a day (such as a 12 oz can of a sweetened soft drink), it would contribute 2,100 calories per week, which could result in approximately 30 pounds of weight gain per year?

My favorite sugar-sweetened-beverage testimony involves my son, Jake. He never really liked soft drinks much, so those weren't an issue, but early in high school, he was on a "Dutch chocolate milk" kick. We talked about all of the extra sugar, fat, and calories in the milk (he knew they were in there!), but he just wanted

MYplace **O** FOR NUTRITION

that sweet, creamy texture and taste, and I basically gave in, knowing that at his growth stage he *really* needed the calcium for his bones, so that took priority with me. He was starting to get a little hefty (but on teen boys that doesn't really show much or at least not right away) and finally just made up his mind one day that he was going cold turkey on the Dutch chocolate milk, switching to skim white milk only. He drank pretty much the same quantity of milk. For most people, this would be a traumatic transition—but not for Jake. He just did it. And, in less than a year, he lost 30 pounds, changing not one other thing about how he ate. He grew to over 6 feet tall and has been at a healthy weight ever since that time.

I cannot stress enough how important it is to *avoid* sugar-sweetened beverages when trying to lose weight and focus on healthy lifestyle changes. If you *do* consume sugar-sweetened beverages, however, do not count them toward your fluid goals on your Live It Tracker.

What About Diet Soft Drinks?

Well, soft drinks with artificial sweeteners don't have all of the excess, empty calories from sugar, it is true. So, yes, they are allowed on the FP4H food plan. However, they also do not contribute any real benefits like the super beverages above, and we want to promote only the *best* choices in FP4H! So, please do not count diet soft drinks toward your daily fluid goals on your Live It Tracker.

Note Regarding Alcoholic Beverages

First Place for Health does not promote or advocate the consumption of alcoholic beverages, but if the choice is made to consume these, the calories provided by them would need to be applied to the daily 100 discretionary calories as mentioned above.

COMMON EXTRAS & ADDITIONS

The condiments and other items listed below do not have any significant nutritional value or benefits and do not contribute to any food group in most cases. We have included this list primarily to help make you aware of how these items contribute to your calorie totals for the day when you add them to your meal plan. Some of them may help you meet your nutrition goals (like a little fat-free salad dressing on your dark leafy green salad, or an occasional serving of sugar-free gelatin to satisfy a sweet tooth), so they are not necessarily bad choices. The FP4H food plan allows for about 100 discretionary calories per day from things like this, but many of these calories may have already been utilized in prior food group choices that have added sugars or fats—so be very careful!

COMMON EXTRAS & ADDITIONS	QUANTITY	TRACKER VALUE	CALORIES
Barbeque Sauce	1 Tbsp		27
Cocktail Sauce	1 Tbsp		21
Coffee Creamer, Dry	1 tsp		11
Coffee Creamer, Liquid	1 Tbsp		20
Cream Cheese, Lite	1 Tbsp		30
Cream Cheese, Fat Free	1 Tbsp		16
Cream/White Sauce	2 Tbsp		91
Gelatin, Sugar Free, Prepared, Fruit Flavor	½ cup		5
Gravy, Prepared from Dry Mix	¼ cup		30
Gravy, Cream/Milk	¼ cup		45
Gravy, Sausage	¼ cup		91
Honey	1 Tbsp		64
Jelly or Jam, Sugar Free (artificial sweetener)	1 Tbsp		18
Jelly or Jam, Low Sugar/All Fruit	1 Tbsp		39
Jelly or Jam, Regular	1 Tbsp		51
Ketchup	1 Tbsp		19
Mustard	1 tsp		3

MYplace ○ FOR NUTRITION

COMMON EXTRAS & ADDITIONS	QUANTITY	TRACKER VALUE	CALORIES
Salad Dressing, Ranch, Fat Free	2 Tbsp		36
Sour Cream, Fat Free	2 Tbsp		20
Sugar, Granulated	1 tsp		16
Sweet and Sour Sauce	1 Tbsp		28
Syrup, Sugar Free	¼ cup		30
Syrup, Maple Flavored, Regular	1 Tbsp		53
Whipped Topping, Non-Dairy, Fat Free	2 Tbsp		15
Whipped Topping, Non-Dairy, Lite	2 Tbsp		20
Whipped Topping, Non-Dairy, Regular	2 Tbsp		30
Half & Half	2 Tbsp	1 tsp fat	40
Sour Cream, Lite	2 Tbsp	1 tsp fat	44
Sour Cream, Regular	2 Tbsp	1 ½ tsp fat	56

PERSONAL FAVORITE EXTRAS

SECTION 1 THE LIVE-IT FOOD PLAN

MYplace O FOR NUTRITION

Recommended Daily Amount of Food from Each Group
(circle the entire column for your level)

GROUP	DAILY CALORIES		
....	1300-1400	1500-1600	1700-1800
Fruits	1.5 – 2 c.	1.5 – 2 c.	1.5 – 2 c.
Vegetables	1.5 – 2 c.	2 – 2.5 c.	2.5 – 3 c.
Grains	5 oz.-eq.	5-6 oz.-eq.	6-7 oz.-eq.
Dairy	2-3 c.	3 c.	3 c.
Protein	4 oz.-eq.	5 oz.-eq.	5-5.5 oz.-eq.
Healthy Oils & Other Fats	4 tsp.	5 tsp.	5 tsp.
Water & Super Beverages*	Women: 9 c. Men: 13 c.	Women: 9 c. Men: 13 c.	Women: 9 c. Men: 13 c.

USING YOUR LIVE IT TRACKER
Live It Tracker

Name: _____

My week at a glance: ○ Great   ○ So-so   ○ Not so great

Activity Level:

○ None   ○ <30 min/day   ○ 30-60 min/day

My activity goal for next week:

○ None   ○ <30 min/day   ○ 30-60 min/day

SECTION 1 THE LIVE-IT FOOD PLAN

1900-2000	2100-2200	2300-2400	2500-2600	2700-2800
2 – 2.5 c.	2 – 2.5 c.	2.5 – 3.5 c.	3.5 – 4.5 c.	3.5 – 4.5 c.
2.5 – 3 c.	3 – 3.5 c.	3.5 – 4.5 c..	4.5 – 5 c.	4.5 – 5 c.
6-7 oz.-eq.	7-8 oz.-eq.	8-9 oz.-eq.	9-10 oz.-eq.	10-11 oz.-eq.
3 c.	3 c.	3 c.	3 c.	3 c.
5.5-6.5 oz.-eq.	6.5-7 oz.-eq.	7-7.5 oz.-eq.	7-7.5 oz.-eq.	7.5-8 oz.-eq.
6 tsp.	6 tsp.	7 tsp.	8 tsp.	8 tsp.
Women: 9 c. Men: 13 c.	Women: 9 c. Men: 13 c.	Women: 9 c. Men: 13 c.	Women: 9 c. Men: 13 c.	Women: 9 c. Men: 13 c.

*May count up to 3 cups caffeinated tea or coffee toward goal

Date: _____ Week # _____

My food goal for next week: _____

_____

_____

_____

MYplace O FOR NUTRITION

Scripture Memory Verse: _____

_____

_____

_____

FOOD CHOICES

Breakfast: _____

_____

Lunch: _____

_____

Dinner: _____

_____

GROUP	FRUITS	VEGETABLES	GRAINS
Estimate Total for Day			
Increase or Decrease?			

SECTION 1 THE LIVE-IT FOOD PLAN

Snacks: _____

_____

PHYSICAL ACTIVITY

Description: _____

_____

_____

Steps/Miles/Minutes: _____

SPIRITUAL ACTIVITY

Description: _____

_____

_____

PROTEIN	DAIRY	HEALTHY OILS & OTHER FATS	WATER & SUPER BEVERAGES

MYplace **O** FOR NUTRITION

The Live It Tracker is a tool by which you can keep a record of your nutrition and physical activities as well as your spiritual disciplines. If you use it consistently, research has shown that you will find success faster, as well as *maintain* that success! I can personally vouch that this tool made *all* the difference in the world to me in my weight-loss journey, because I knew I had to be honest and tell someone what I was actually doing—no more hiding!

Completing your Live It Tracker involves the following steps:

1. Write your name, start date of the tracker, week number (refer to your Bible study for that), and your current activity level (circle one of the choices provided). Be sure that the start date of the tracker is the day your group *meets* so that it will be completely finished on the day *prior* to your next group meeting, ready to turn in to your leader!

2. Write two goals for yourself at the beginning of each week when you start a new tracker, one of which pertains to your food choices and the other to your activity. For example, a food goal might be to "eat at least 1 ½ cups fruit each day" or "limit desserts to two nights this week." An activity goal might be to "take the stairs every day at work."

3. Write the Scripture memory verse for that week on the lines provided. This will help you learn the verse and will serve as a reminder for you to work on memorizing the verse throughout the week every time you look at your tracker.

4. Find your recommended calorie range in the Recommended Daily Amount of Food from Each Group table. *Circle* that entire column of the table.

5. List your food choices on the lines provided for all meals and snacks every day. At the *end* of each day, estimate your total for each group and write these values on the row that says "Estimate your total."

6. Assess your food quantity by using up and down arrows. Indicate if you need to eat more or less of each food group on the row that says "Increase or Decrease?" Just draw a dash if you met your goal and do not need to increase or decrease the number of servings.

SECTION 1 **THE LIVE-IT FOOD PLAN**

7. Provide a description for your spiritual activities (reading your Bible, practicing your Scripture memory verse, doing your FP4H Bible study for that day, contacting a group member, attending worship service, etc.). Feel free to abbreviate! For instance, on my tracker I just write "FPBS" for doing the Bible Study, "MV" for working on the verse, and "contacted __" (initials of person I contacted that day).

8. Provide a description of the physical activities for the day (for example: "walked 3 miles," "walked 10,235 steps," or "lifted weights for 20 minutes"). Be sure to include the number of steps, miles, or minutes for your physical activities. In my group, we convert everything to "miles" using the conversion information in the back of each Bible study. Then, we mark our progress on the 100-mile chart inside the back cover of the study each week. When someone reaches each 50-mile increment, we give them some sort of small (non-food) reward!

9. At the *end* of each week, assess how you did in achieving your personal goals and basic goals of FP4H. Rate your week by checking "Great," "So-so," or "Not so great."

Note: You might also want to consider the use of online programs or apps for your mobile device to assist you with tracking your food (e.g., "MyFitnessPal," "Lose It"). Please print the records weekly (or share online with your leader) and turn in your paper tracker with the other information written in (estimated daily total of each food group, spiritual activity) that is not included on the online version, to stay accountable in all areas.

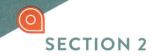

SECTION 2

Primary Session Wellness Worksheets

Practicing Mindfulness

Many of our not-so-healthy eating habits have developed over a long period of time. Very often we eat not because we are hungry but out of habit, in response to various triggers in our environment.

Let's take a look at some examples of things that could have been an influence during our childhood:

1. Food used as a reward for good behavior
   ("If you are still and quiet during church, we will go get ice cream later!")

2. Food used as a reward for good performance
   ("Since you made all As on your report card, we will go get a kid's meal at _____ after school today!")

3. Food used as a punishment
   ("You behaved terribly at the grocery store—no dessert for you tonight!")

4. The "clean your plate" mentality
   ("All those starving children in Africa would love to have that..." or "I would have never complained if I had something that good to eat when I was your age!")

5. Patterning eating behaviors after significant adults in our lives
   (For instance, if we always saw our parents eating straight out of a bag of chips or eating ice cream every night before bed, then we would probably be more likely to do that ourselves.)

SECTION 2 PRIMARY SESSION WELLNESS WORKSHEETS

Can you relate to any of these? Do any others come to mind? _____

_____

_____

_____

_____

_____

This is not to say that our families meant to do us any harm by doing these things—they are actually very common behaviors and are usually intended to help! The problem is that, over time, we have learned to give food a value that it really doesn't have. We may have also tried to use food as a medicine or remedy for certain situations. Maybe you have eaten to:

1. Deal with stress

2. Avoid/put off difficult tasks

3. Deal with difficult people

4. Comfort yourself in good or bad times

5. Prevent boredom

Any other reasons you can think of? _____

_____

_____

_____

_____

_____

_____

MYplace O FOR NUTRITION

Obviously, eating food cannot fix any of those situations, can it? It might make us feel better for a very short period of time, but those situations are still there when the food is completely out of your system! (Note: You will have the opportunity to delve more into emotional eating in the *My Place for Discovery* book.)

"If you accept that your habits or behaviors have contributed to weight gain, then it makes sense to use an approach that goes beyond just reducing calories to lose weight. To make permanent changes in your body weight, you must change the behaviors that caused the problems in the first place."[2]

Behavior modification therapy has been used for over 35 years as an approach to change life habits such as smoking, overeating, and stress management. It is now accepted as a *vital* part of any weight-control program and is best if combined with a calorie-controlled eating plan (like the "Live-it") and increased physical activity.

KEEPING A FOOD & EXERCISE JOURNAL

Research has shown time and time again that this is the *single most effective* behavior in successful weight loss/maintenance. If you are more *aware* of what you are eating and have to record it somewhere, you just end up eating less! See "Using Your Live It Tracker" in the preceding pages for instructions on how to complete these forms. In addition to tracking, below are several behavior modifications you can use in various environments to help you reach your weight goals:[3]

Home Environment

1. Eat *only* while sitting down at the kitchen or dining room table (*not* while watching TV, reading, cooking, talking on the phone, standing in front of the refrigerator, or working on the computer!).

2. Keep unhealthy (or tempting) foods out the house or out of sight. (It is best not to buy them, but if you must, keep them in a high cabinet, not in clear containers.)

3. Keep cut-up/washed fruits and vegetables in the front of the refrigerator.

4. Keep *pre-portioned* healthy snacks on hand (whole-grain crackers, nuts—buy bulk and pre-portion them yourself to save money).

Work Environment

1. Don't eat at your desk.

2. Take a healthy lunch and healthy snacks for between meals.

3. Keep water with you to drink during the day.

4. Go for a walk during breaks.

5. Avoid trigger areas (such as staff break rooms with donuts, or a convenience store on your way to/from work).

6. If you work around food, plan in advance what you will eat.

7. Don't work through meal times (skipping meals can slow down your metabolism over time *and* result in overeating at the next meal—a double whammy!).

8. For celebrations, offer to bring a healthy item, and if you choose to eat other items, eat only very small amounts. Only fill your (small) plate *one* time!

Mealtime/Eating Environment

1. Serve your plate at the stove or kitchen counter, portioning carefully, before sitting down at the table.

2. Use smaller plates, bowls, and glasses—a smaller portion will look large when it is in a little dish.

3. Drink a glass of water before starting to eat.

4. Avoid/limit high-calorie condiments.

5. Eat slowly—it takes 10 to 15 minutes for your stomach to send a message to your brain that it is full.

6. Take small bites and chew your food well.

7. Put your eating utensil down on the table between bites, and take a sip of water.

8. Do not cut your food all at one time, but only as needed.

9. Stop eating at points during the meal to reflect and converse.

10. Freeze or refrigerate leftovers in individual portions.

Shopping

1. Don't shop for food when you are hungry or tired.

2. Always shop with a list.

3. Don't taste test in the store.

4. Read/compare food labels for best nutrition.

5. Stay closer to the perimeter of the store (versus in the center) as much as possible.

Restaurants

1. Don't arrive hungry—eat something light before the meal (for example: a piece of fruit or a cup of yogurt, or any food that you probably won't have access to at the restaurant but that you *need* to eat that day).

SECTION 2 PRIMARY SESSION WELLNESS WORKSHEETS

2. Check out the restaurant menu online and make choices ahead of time.

3. Do *not* skip other meals in the day.

4. Order a la carte rather than full meals.

5. With higher-calorie dishes, share or box half to take home.

6. Ask for salad dressings, gravies, and sauces on the side and dip fork in before eating, rather than pouring on food.

7. Drink water or other no-calorie beverages.

Holidays

1. Have lower-calorie and healthy foods/beverages on hand at all times (for yourself *and* guests).

2. Keep tempting foods out of sight until actual service (prevents nibbling!).

3. Allow yourself one planned treat per day.

4. Don't skip meals to save up for holiday meals/parties.

5. Don't forget to continue to make time for exercise!

"Do not conform to the pattern of this world, but be transformed by the renewing of your mind. Then you will be able to test and approve what God's will is—His good, pleasing and perfect will."

—Romans 12:1-2, NIV

Your past life experiences have helped create the pattern you follow—pray for God's help to become more mindful and transform it into a pattern more pleasing to Him!

MYplace O FOR NUTRITION

MINDFULNESS ACTIVITY

List at least five behavior-modification tips from the above that you plan to begin using this week:

1. _____

_____

_____

2. _____

_____

_____

3. _____

_____

_____

4. _____

_____

_____

5. _____

_____

_____

EATING HEALTHY WHEN EATING OUT

I remember that when I was a child, eating in a restaurant was a rare treat reserved for very special occasions. It probably had something to do with the fact that there were six children in my family and my parents were raising us on a pastor's salary!

Today, recent statistics show that the average American adult buys a meal or snack from a restaurant 5.8 times a week, and more than 30% of children eat fast food on any given day. We now spend more than half of our food budget eating out[4], so I think that it is safe to say that most of us eat out *a lot* more now than we did growing up. Whether the reason is time, convenience, variety, value, or simply entertainment/socializing, we are pulling into the drive-thru or stopping for a meal away from home on a regular basis.

People who are trying to eat healthier meals are presented with mind-boggling choices and temptations, but believe it or not, you *can* dine out without blowing it; you just need to know how. The keys to success are having a plan for healthy eating, sticking with it, and exercising your rights as a consumer by asking for exactly what you want.

Many fast-food restaurant chains actually provide calorie information on their menu boards now, so that can be a big help in narrowing down your choices in that arena. Also, due to more health-conscious patrons, many sit-down restaurant chains now have a "lower calorie" entrée section on their menus (usually between 400 and 600 calories) or a special symbol designating those items.

Those chains that don't display any nutrition information on a board or menu usually have it available on their websites. I have found it very helpful to go online and look at nutrition information before I go to a restaurant. In doing so, I can actually make my choice in advance, when I don't feel quite so pressed for time. This also helps me set my mind so that I don't feel as influenced by the multitude of choices or the recommendations from others eating with me. I often even go ahead and record my chosen meal on my FP4H food records *before* I eat so that I am more likely to stick with it.

As available as nutrition information is for chain restaurants, however, not all restaurants provide this service to consumers. A few behavior-modification tips were given in the restaurant section of the "Practicing Mindfulness" wellness worksheet, but here are a few more, especially for when you don't have access to specific nutrition information:

MYplace ○ FOR NUTRITION

- Try to avoid all-you-can-eat buffet restaurants, especially in your early efforts to control your portions. These are super-tempting, confusing and often create a feeling that you want to get your money's worth, so you just tend to eat too much.

- Start off with a salad with a fat-free/light dressing (served on the side) or a broth-based vegetable soup. This will help you get some healthy vegetables *and* curb your appetite so that you are not as tempted to overeat later. Ask them to leave off cheese/croutons/crackers to save more calories/grain servings for later.

- Ask if you may substitute steamed/grilled vegetables, fruit, or a salad for fried side items.

- Ask the person taking your order to leave off sauces/condiments on meats/ sandwiches (or serve them on the side) so that you can control the amount eaten. This especially applies to cream sauces/gravies, mayonnaise/regular salad dressings, butter and margarine, since they are heavy on fat and calories—even in small amounts.

- Ask if they can split the entrée ahead of time (or just bring you a carry-out container with your entrée) so that you can divide it immediately to take half home for another meal.

- Ask them to hold the salt or use salt-free seasoning.

- Restaurants usually list meat as the raw weight *before* cooking (which makes them look more generous!), and meats generally lose about one quarter of that weight during the cooking process. Therefore, a 6-oz sirloin steak would end up counting as 4 oz of protein, a 9-oz steak as 7 oz., etc. If the meat weight isn't listed on the menu, another way to estimate your portion is that a 3-oz serving looks like the size/thickness of a deck of playing cards.

- When estimating amounts for other food items, think of these visual cues: 1 cup looks about like a baseball or computer mouse; ½ cup looks like it would fit in a regular size cupcake wrapper or a level ice cream scoop; 1 tablespoon would be like an iPhone wall charger; 1 teaspoon would be like a dice.

SECTION 2 PRIMARY SESSION WELLNESS WORKSHEETS

○ When eating out with family and friends, tell them in advance that you plan to eat healthy. If you know that a meal will be relatively high in calories and fat, choose healthier foods during the rest of the day and be more physically active.

When you ask for foods to be served differently than listed on the menu, you may feel like you are being difficult or picky—but you are *not*! You are being proactive and are making healthy choices for your physical body, God's temple—something that is definitely worth your effort. Most restaurants accommodate special requests these days without any real problem, and sometimes what you are asking for (like leaving something off) even costs the restaurant less money or time in preparation!

Menu Terminology Clues

Menus are full of food clues, if you know what to look for. Start choosing more items prepared using healthier cooking methods. Below is a list of terms that may be helpful:

BETTER CHOICES	CAUTION CHOICES
GENERAL	**GENERAL**
• Baked	• Deep fried
• Broiled	• Pan fried
• Roasted	• Sautéed (*using a lot of butter or oil*)
• Braised	• Prime
• Poached	• Casserole
• Steamed	• Breaded
• Stir-fried	• Cream sauce
• Grilled	
• Sautéed (*with broth, cooking spray, or minimal oil*)	
ASIAN	**ASIAN**
• Jum (*poached*)	• Duck
• Kow (*roasted*)	• Egg rolls
• Shu (*barbecued*)	• Fried or Crispy
• Steamed dumplings (*rice, chicken, shrimp*)	• Peanuts or Cashews
• Water chestnuts	• Tempura
• Sushi (*depending on dipping sauce*)	• Wonton

MYplace O FOR NUTRITION

BETTER CHOICES

ITALIAN

- Cacciatore *(means "with stewed vegetables")*
- Marsala *(wine sauce)*
- Marinara *(tomato-based sauce)*
- Minestrone
- Primavera *(means "with fresh vegetables")*
- Red sauce
- White clam sauce
- Crushed tomatoes
- Sun-dried tomatoes
- Lightly sautéed
- Whole-wheat pasta
- Whole-wheat pizza crust

MEXICAN/TEX-MEX

- Asada *(means "grilled")*
- Fajitas
- Picante sauce
- Salsa
- Salsa verde *(green sauce)*
- Veracruz or Ranchero *(tomato-based)*
- Steamed or soft corn tortillas
- Tortilla soup
- Bean soup
- Red sauce
- Enchilada sauce
- Pico de gallo
- Charro beans
- Black beans

CAUTION CHOICES

ITALIAN

- Alfredo
- Creama *(means "cream-based sauce")*
- Fritta or Fritto *(fried)*
- Parmigiana *(breaded & deep fried)*
- Some cheese & meat-filled pastas *(such as ravioli, manicotti, or cannelloni—be sure to check nutrition information online if available!)*
- Pesto *(watch amount—healthy oil but 1 Tbsp can have 60-80 calories)*

MEXICAN/TEX-MEX

- Chili con queso *(cheese sauce)*
- Chorizo *(sausage)*
- Fried or Crispy
- Sour cream
- Refried *(often with lard)*
- Tortilla chips *(watch amount—healthy oil and whole grain but 5-7 chips have about 100 calories)*
- Guacamole *(healthy oil but watch amount—1/4 cup has about 100 calories)*

United States Healthful Food Council, http://ushfc.org.

SECTION 2 PRIMARY SESSION WELLNESS WORKSHEETS

RESTAURANT ACTIVITY

In the following table, list the restaurants where you dine most often and your usual choices at that restaurant. What foods would be better choices?

RESTAURANT	USUAL CHOICES (be specific)	BETTER CHOICES

MYplace ○ FOR NUTRITION

UNDERSTANDING NUTRITION LABELS

First of all, I want to emphasize that *many* of the healthy foods we need to be eating don't even *have* a nutrition label! Choices such as fresh fruits and vegetables and fresh, unprocessed meats should be staples of our diet. However, I realize that some really healthy foods are only available as packaged items (most of us don't bake our own whole-grain cereals or crackers from scratch, for instance). Therefore, some guidance is needed in making the healthiest choices in the processed-food arena. Grocery stores are full of frozen meals, canned soups, dried pasta mixes, packaged snack foods, and more. These foods *might* save us a little time, but they can also be very high in calories and have harmful saturated and/or trans fats, added sugars, and sodium—all of which can sabotage our healthy lifestyle efforts if we are not careful.

Don't be fooled or confused by nutrition claims on the front labels of pre-packaged foods. These claims are regulated to a certain degree, but the easiest, wisest thing you can do is flip the package over and look at two things: (1) the nutrition facts label, and (2) the ingredients listing.

The Nutrition Facts label has undergone many regulatory changes over the years. Below is a diagram of the current label (on the left) and the new label (final rule published in May 2016), currently scheduled to be implemented no later than January 2020 for larger food manufacturing companies.[5]

Note: The label images are meant for illustrative purposes to show how the new Nutrition Facts label might look compared to the old label. Both labels represent fictional products. When the original hypothetical label was developed in 2014 (the image on the left-hand side), added sugars was not yet proposed so the "original" label shows 1g of sugar as an example. The image created for the "new" label (shown on the right-hand side) lists 12g total sugar and 10g added sugar to give an example of how added sugars would be broken out with a % Daily Value.

SECTION 2 PRIMARY SESSION WELLNESS WORKSHEETS

INGREDIENTS

Ingredients are usually listed just below the nutrition facts label, and they must be listed in order from the *greatest amount* included (by weight) in the food or drink to the *least* amount. For example, if you see sugar (or one of its other names, such as corn syrup) listed at the beginning or close to the beginning of the ingredients list, then you know that the food or drink you're looking at is relatively high in sugar. Another example might be a canned vegetable soup with the first ingredient water, second ingredient carrots, third ingredient tomatoes, etc. This would mean that the soup may actually be a decent choice, since some sort of modified food starch isn't listed before the vegetables. In other words, based on this list, you can make an educated guess about which food groups the product includes. The bottom line? Look for products with the fewest ingredients—and the ones you can pronounce and recognize as foods!

SERVING SIZE

The Food and Drug Administration (FDA) determines the serving size described on the food labels of many foods. This information is vital in understanding the remaining numbers on the label, since everything on the label is based on that portion size. The new label will require manufacturers to list a portion size that reflects what people currently eat, rather than what the companies decide seems reasonable. For example, a serving of ice cream is currently listed as ½ cup but will be shown as 2/3 cup on the future label. A serving of soda was 8 oz but will now be 12 oz (since this is the most typical can size). This was a very controversial change but the bottom line remains the same—the calories and other nutrients are for *that* portion size. Therefore, if you eat *twice* that portion size, you would double that information to get the correct nutrient information for what you eat. If you eat half of that portion size, you would divide it by two, and so on.

CALORIES

Calories are a unit of measurement for the amount of food energy provided by a particular food. Our body uses calories like our vehicles use fuel. However, if we consume too much fuel for our metabolism/activity level, our bodies store the extra as fat. On the new label, the total calorie count is to be highlighted in large, bold print rather than being in the same type size as the other nutrition information, to help consumers be more aware of this information.

MYplace O FOR NUTRITION

PERCENTAGE DAILY VALUE

(%DV) Percentage Daily Values are based on a 2,000-calorie diet and are to be used as a frame of reference only. Your daily values may be higher or lower, depending on your individual needs. However, this section does give you some valuable information regarding the proportion of nutrients in a food and whether a food is high or low in nutrients. Use this information not only to help you limit those nutrients you want to cut back on (saturated fat, trans fat, sodium) but also to increase those nutrients you need to consume in greater amounts (fiber, calcium, iron, potassium, vitamin D).

For example, you may be trying to choose a good whole-grain breakfast cereal. The first one you look at shows whole wheat as the first ingredient and it has 150 calories per cup with 2 grams of fiber. The one next to it also has whole wheat as the first ingredient, but it has 165 calories with 7 grams of fiber. I would go with the second choice myself, to help me reach my daily fiber goal (at least 25 grams), and not worry a lot about the 15 additional calories.

On the new label, manufacturers must declare the actual amount, in addition to Percent Daily Value, of vitamin D, calcium, iron and potassium. They can *voluntarily* declare the gram amount for other vitamins and minerals. Vitamins A and C will no longer be required on labels, since deficiencies of these vitamins are rare nowadays. I am personally happy for the new vitamin D information. Though I get plenty of milk products in my diet, since I am not out in the sun a lot, I actually need to add vitamin D-rich foods to keep my levels within normal limits for bone health—and many middle-aged and older adults face this same challenge. Potassium has been added because of its role in helping lower blood pressure.

TOTAL FAT, SATURATED FAT, & TRANS FAT

Total fat is provided in grams and % Daily Value. For reference purposes, 5 grams of fat is about one teaspoon and provides about 45 calories (regardless of the source). Based on research that shows that the type of fat is more important than the amount, the "Calories from Fat" line will disappear on the new label. However, the new label will continue the requirement for the subcategories of "saturated fat" and "trans fat," which is very helpful information. Saturated fat is one of the worst things for your health, increasing your risk for heart disease. Trans fat has been shown to be even *more* dangerous for the same reason, so you would like for this to be zero grams. Most food manufacturers are now aware that this type of fat is not acceptable and have stopped using it, but you may find it occasionally. Therefore, keep a close watch on this section of the label when choosing convenience foods. (Note: The types of fats will be discussed further in the "Preventing Heart Disease" wellness worksheet, so stay tuned!)

CHOLESTEROL

Cholesterol is found only in animal products, with the highest sources in organ meats, shellfish and egg yolks. Though this information will still be required on the new label, much new research is showing us that dietary cholesterol does not have the same detrimental effects on our blood cholesterol as do saturated and trans fats. However, the jury is still out to some degree, so the dietary cholesterol information is provided, and many health experts still recommend consuming fewer than 300 mg per day for the best possible prevention of heart disease. Our bodies actually make all of the cholesterol we need—so we don't have to get it from food!

SODIUM

High sodium intake is linked to high blood pressure/hypertension, though research shows that some people are more salt sensitive than others. However, it is widely accepted by health experts that we *all* tend to consume much more sodium than we need, primarily because of the multitude of processed foods we eat. It is recommended in the latest U.S. Dietary Guidelines and by the Institute of Medicine that our daily consumption of sodium not exceed 2,300 mg. Intakes over this limit are considered to be harmful to your health. A teaspoon of table salt has about 2,400 mg of sodium. Please pay attention to this section of the label when you are choosing convenience foods—especially frozen entrées and canned soups—or you may get half (or more) of the daily recommendation in only *one* serving of *one* item!

TOTAL CARBOHYDRATES & FIBER

Carbohydrates are found naturally in grains, fruits, vegetables, and milk products. They are our brain's preferred source of energy and are necessary for health. The FP4H Live It plan is designed so that about half of your daily calories are coming from carbohydrates. Carbohydrates are absorbed and digested very quickly by our bodies, at least compared to proteins and fats, which take longer to break

MYplace O FOR NUTRITION

down. Therefore, carbohydrates become glucose in the blood relatively quickly, so diabetics are especially interested in this section of the label. About 15 grams of carbohydrate is the amount found in 1 oz of a grain product or ½ cup of fruit, which is helpful information when trying to figure out how much to count a convenience product on your FP4H tracker (or how much insulin to take, if you are a diabetic).

Health experts tell us that the majority of our carbohydrates need to come from complex sources, what many people just call "good" carbs. Complex carbohydrates are the ones that are relatively higher in fiber content and take a little longer to break down to glucose, such as those found in whole grains and fresh fruits and vegetables. The daily adult goal for fiber intake is 21 to 38 grams depending on your age and gender. When you choose whole grains, fresh fruits and vegetables often (as the FP4H food plan recommends), this will not be a difficult goal to reach. (Note: More detailed information on fiber, including the different types, is included in the "Fiber & Gluten Facts" wellness worksheet.)

Unfortunately, most people consume too many of the not-so-good or simple (not complex) carbohydrates, sometimes not really understanding where the carbohydrates are coming from. Therefore, the new label format requires that manufacturers break out the "added sugars" so that we will be informed about how many grams of carbohydrate occurred naturally in the food and how many were added in the form of table sugar, corn syrup, or other additives. Currently, the label just says "sugars," which actually includes things like the natural sugar in milk (lactose) and in fruits (fructose). Though these are technically simple sugars, being naturally occurring in the foods God has provided for us, they are definitely healthier for consumption than *added* sugars.

To explain a little further: A cup of plain fat-free milk has about 12 grams of sugar (lactose)—but this is a natural, healthy, *good* choice for a high-calcum dairy product, with only about 90 calories and no fat—not harmful. On the other hand, if you drink a cup of Dutch chocolate milk, it has about 210 calories and 27 grams of sugar, plus 8 grams of fat (5 of which are saturated). Since you now know that 12 of those grams of sugar were in the milk naturally, you know that 15 of them were added. Four grams of sugar is equal to about a teaspoon of sugar—so we are talking about almost 4 teaspoons in this one cup of chocolate milk. The new label will take the guesswork and complicated calculations out, so I am pretty excited about this new requirement!

PROTEIN

Proteins function as building blocks for bones, muscles, skin, and blood, so they are vital to the smooth and healthy operation of our temples. A one-ounce portion of meat has about 7 grams of protein, one cup of milk has about 8 grams, and most grains even have 2-3 grams per ounce. Keep these facts in mind when trying to figure out how to count a convenience food on your Live It Tracker. For example, if you choose a frozen chicken pasta entrée that appears to be mostly pasta (judging by the ingredient list and visual cues), and you see only 4 grams of protein on the nutrition facts label, then there is probably not enough meat in that choice to provide even one ounce for helping meet your protein group needs for the day.

LABEL ACTIVITY

Go to your food cabinet, choose a processed food, and answer the following (or just write n/a if not provided):

Brand/Name of Food: _____

Serving Size: _____

Servings Per Container:_____

Calories:_____

Fat (grams): _____Carbohydrate (grams): _____

Dietary Fiber (grams): _____Sugars (grams): _____

Added Sugars (grams):_____Protein (grams): _____

MYplace O FOR NUTRITION

LABEL ACTIVITY

Do any of the vitamins or minerals listed (calcium, iron, vitamin D, potassium, vitamin A, vitamin C, or others) have 20% or more of the Daily Value? If so, which ones? _____

_____

First 3 ingredients listed: _____

_____

_____

Based on the ingredient listing and nutrition facts panel, which FP4H food groups do you think this food may contribute to, if any? Check all that may apply:

_____ Fruit   _____ Protein

_____ Vegetable   _____ Dairy

_____ Grain   _____ Healthy Oils/Other Fats

SECTION 2 PRIMARY SESSION WELLNESS WORKSHEETS

RECIPE TRANSFORMATION TACTICS

I love to cook! Like my three older sisters, I learned to cook from my mother, often standing on a chair beside her in the kitchen. She always said she wanted all of her daughters to learn to cook, because she didn't learn until after she got married—and she *really* wished she had some training before that! Therefore, the very first badge I earned in my Brownie troop (the youngest division of Girl Scouts) was the cooking badge, and I proudly attached it to my uniform sash at the age of 7 or 8, thanks to Mama! My love for cooking definitely led to my interest in nutrition, which eventually landed me in the profession of dietetics. On a side note, my mother (Mary) has been a member of my FP4H groups for many years, having lost over 30 pounds on the program and kept it off for many years now. Interestingly enough, she is best buddies with another senior adult member of my group (Bunny), who just happens to be my very first Home Economics teacher from high school. Bunny experienced about the same weight loss as Mama in another FP4H group many years ago but has been coming to our group for quite some time now, also maintaining her healthy weight. It is truly a joy and a blessing to have both of them there—they have very sweet spirits and bring much experience, encouragement and wisdom to the group!

Maybe you have lots of cookbooks on your shelves like I do. I lost count at 75 or so! I have collected them for years, and many friends have given them to me as gifts. Some of the cookbooks are fancy, beautiful low-fat or diabetic volumes, given to me because of my profession, but I actually don't use those very much. The ones that are on the easiest-to-reach shelf in my kitchen are the good old

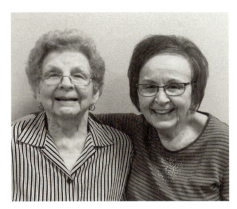

church and club cookbooks, collections from the best cooks in the bunch. The book I use most often is held together with a rubber band! Did I give up my favorite recipes from these books after joining FP4H? Absolutely not. Remember, First Place for Health is not a diet but a "Live It"—so this worksheet is to help you modify the recipes you already

MYplace O FOR NUTRITION

love so that you can continue to lose weight and/or maintain your weight loss in the years to come without feeling cheated out of anything. And if you find a new recipe you want to try out from a magazine or website, this information will help you do that in a healthier way!

You can make almost any recipe healthier with just a few simple changes. Use the following tips to help turn your recipes into healthier alternatives:

Start with the Basics

- Look at the ingredient list to see if there are any obvious ways to cut calories, fat, sugar, or sodium. Often you can achieve this by simply choosing the lighter versions of various products—such as light sour cream, light cream cheese, 2% cheese, lower-sodium soups, extra-lean ground beef, turkey bacon, fat-free milk, and so forth. Sometimes you can just use less of the original ingredient and make a huge difference!

- Make changes gradually to learn what works best. Changing ingredients can affect taste, texture, and appearance, so you may have to do some experimenting. For instance, a cheese ball appetizer or cream pie using fat-free cream cheese alone will most likely end up a spread instead of a ball, or a goo instead of a slice-able pie, so you might want to go with the one-third less fat version, or a combination of regular and fat free, or add another stabilizing ingredient, such as a small portion of pudding mix, to thicken it up.

- Remember, this is the Live It plan, so for that extra-special occasion when you don't want to change a super-special favorite recipe ("passed down for generations," etc.), just serve a small portion and don't go back for seconds.

Cooking Tips for Cutting Facts

- Use a nonstick cooking spray or a spritz of olive oil, or even small amounts of broth or fruit juice to sauté vegetables or pan fry meats instead of butter or margarine.

- Limit meat portions in your entrée recipes to 3 ounces or less per serving.

SECTION 2 PRIMARY SESSION WELLNESS WORKSHEETS

You can make up for the reduced portion size and increase nutrition by adding more grains, vegetables, or legumes. Or go meatless and use beans, lentils, peas, or soy products instead of the meat, which virtually eliminates all of the saturated fat.Use meats trimmed of visible fat, and drain fat from meat during/after cooking. Rinse cooked ground meats with hot water to remove much of the fat.

- Refrigerate broths, soups and stews before serving. Remove the layer of fat that forms at the top and hardens after cooling, and then reheat the broth.

- Egg substitutes or two egg whites may be substituted for a whole egg to cut calories, fat, and cholesterol, but remember that whole eggs used in moderation are OK as part of an overall healthy diet.

- If a recipe calls for butter or margarine, try using half of that amount of vegetable oil in its place (example: substitute ½ cup canola oil for 1 cup butter).

- In recipes calling for cheese, use 1/3 to ½ of what the recipe calls for and/or use low-fat cheese (3-5 grams fat per ounce). Choose a sharp cheese for more flavor.

- Replace some of the fat in baked goods with fruit purées such as applesauce or "baby food" fruits like bananas, peaches or prunes. Use ½ cup of the purée in place of 1 cup of butter, shortening or oil. Don't get rid of all of the fat though. You will probably need to add 1-2 tablespoons of the fat to achieve the best results.

- Use low-fat or nonfat cream cheese, sour cream, yogurt, mayonnaise, and salad dressing instead of the full-fat regular versions.

- In recipes calling for nuts, cut the amount down to ½ or even ¼ of the amount called for. If the crunch is all you want, you can even substitute a few tablespoons of a whole-grain cereal like Grape Nuts.

MYplace O FOR NUTRITION

Cooking Tips for Cutting Sugar

O Try using ¼ to ½ less sugar than what the recipe calls for—you probably won't even notice the difference, and this will really lower the empty calorie level. Learn to make special treats with fruits, such as fruit and yogurt parfaits or smoothies, frozen fruit pops, frozen bananas, and trail mix.

O Experiment using fruit juice concentrates instead of sugar. Remember to reduce the overall liquid in the recipe if you do this.

O You may choose to substitute artificial or natural low-calorie sweeteners for all or part of the sugar in a recipe, but remember that they do not have all of the same chemical properties that sugar does, so experimentation is usually needed for best results. (Note: See the "Preventing and Managing Diabetes" Wellness Worksheet for more detailed information about this topic.)

Cooking Tips for Cutting Sodium

O Add flavor to vegetables, meats, poultry, and fish by using herbs and spices instead of salt or high-sodium seasonings or sauces.

O Choose lower-sodium versions of purchased soups, broths, and sauces. Better yet, make your own broth for soups and use minimal salt in preparation—it will probably still be much less sodium that any you could buy and it will taste better!

O Eliminate or cut the salt in half for most of your recipes. Many seasoning packets in convenience-food pasta or rice mixes are very high in sodium. Just use ½ or less of the packet, or just don't use it at all, and substitute with your own herbs and spices.

O Drain and rinse canned vegetables with water to wash away extra sodium.

Cooking Tips for Adding Nutrition

O Increase fiber by substituting whole-wheat flour, oats, or whole-grain cornmeal for some of the white flour in recipes. Substitute with whole-wheat flour ½ of the white flour in the recipe, or substitute 1/3 of white flour with oats.

SECTION 2 PRIMARY SESSION WELLNESS WORKSHEETS

○ Keep the peels on fruits and vegetables such as potatoes, carrots, and apples.

○ Add extra vegetables or legumes, or whole grains such as brown rice, whole-wheat pasta, or quinoa, to soups, sauces, salads, and casseroles. On pasta and rice dishes, you might want to start with ½ white and ½ whole grain for a less-drastic change, especially with children.

○ Add fruits such as fresh/dried berries or mandarin orange slices to green salads.

○ Add small amounts of chopped or sliced nuts to salads or baked goods.

○ Top a baked potato with steamed, fresh, or stir-fried vegetables.

○ Replace half or more of the iceberg lettuce in salads with dark green varieties like romaine. Add baby spinach and chopped kale for even more of a nutrition boost.

RECIPE ACTIVITY

After reviewing the suggested modifications for various ingredients, head to your kitchen and grab a cookbook or locate a recipe online to practice making the changes. List the name of the recipe below and the ingredients, then make suggestions for healthy substitutions/additions:

RECIPE NAME: _____

INGREDIENTS:	HEALTHIER SUBSTITION (OR ADDITION):

MYplace O FOR NUTRITION

HABITS FOR A HEALTHY HEART

Did you know that heart disease is the leading cause of death in the United States for both men and women? Cardiovascular issues affect people of every age, ethnicity, and background. About 610,000 Americans die from heart disease each year—that's 1 in every 4 deaths. In the U.S., someone has a heart attack about every 42 seconds, and each *minute* someone in the United States dies from a heart-related event. Coronary Artery Disease (CAD) is the most common type of heart disease, killing about 365,000 people in 2014. It is caused by plaque build-up in the wall of the arteries that supply blood to the heart (called coronary arteries). Plaque is made up of cholesterol deposits, and the build-up of these causes the inside of the arteries to narrow over time, creating problems with blood flow to the heart. This process is called atherosclerosis.[6] This condition can worsen to the point that the blood flow to the heart can be completely blocked or the plaque can rupture, causing a heart attack. If this occurs in the arteries to the *brain*, a stroke can result. While a heart attack or stroke can occur suddenly, in many cases, atherosclerosis develops as a result of many years of unhealthy choices.

This topic has a special place in my personal priorities because heart disease runs in my family on my father's side. I have had some first cousins who died with heart attack and stroke in their 40s and early 50s. In March 1995, Daddy was making a pastoral visit to a member of his congregation at a Little Rock hospital, and while walking back to the car after the visit, he experienced some dizziness and severe weakness. He made it to the car and drove back to Searcy (about 50 miles), straight to his doctor's office. They checked him out and he ended up in the same Little Rock hospital he had just been visiting—scheduled for heart bypass surgery. The surgery procedure was scary but successful. As is typical following any heart surgery, he and my mother received a lot of patient education regarding healthy behaviors he needed to adopt to prevent further episodes. Daddy was overweight and didn't have a very healthy lifestyle up to this point, but things changed drastically

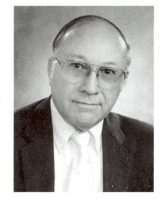

after that surgery. With his blessing and encouragement, I started my very first FP4H group soon after this experience, and he supported his "little girl" by being one of those first 28 members. Daddy followed the FP4H food plan, exercised regularly, and lost over 30 pounds in that first session! He continued to lose weight in the subsequent session, his cholesterol levels improved, and he adopted a pretty healthy lifestyle overall. I firmly believe that it was because of those changes that we were blessed to have him with us for another 15 years.

THE 10 MAJOR RISK FACTORS

There are now ten major risk factors for heart disease, according to the American Heart Association.[7] The more factors a person has, the greater the risk of heart attack and stroke. Notice that the first three are factors that cannot be changed, but the rest (thankfully!) can be avoided by making lifestyle changes.

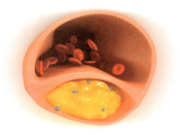

1. Increasing age. More than 83% of people who die of coronary heart disease are age 65 or older.

What is your age?_____

2. Gender. Men are more likely to have heart attacks than women, and they typically have them earlier in life. Women's death rates from heart disease increase after menopause; however, it's not as great as men's.

What is your gender?_____

3. Heredity (including race). Your risk is higher if you have a family history of heart disease. In addition, heart disease is higher among African Americans, Mexican Americans, Native Americans, native Hawaiians, and some Asian Americans. Note that most people with a strong family history have one or more other risk factors.

MYplace O FOR NUTRITION

Do you have a family history of heart disease? _____

4. Smoking. A smoker's risk of developing heart disease is two to four times that of a nonsmoker. Secondhand smoke also increases your risk. A smoker is much more likely to die when a heart attack or stroke occurs than a nonsmoker. If you smoke, make every possible effort to quit.

Are you currently a smoker, or are you exposed to frequent secondhand smoke?

_____

5. Abnormal cholesterol levels. The risk of heart disease rises as the total and LDL (bad) cholesterol levels increase. The risk of heart disease also rises as HDL (good) cholesterol levels *decrease*. High triglycerides may also increase your risk.

If your numbers are in the high or borderline-high range and you have two or more other risk factors, you may be greatly adding to your risk of heart attack or stroke. Talk to your doctor. Treatment and prevention alway involve lifestyle changes, such

WHAT ARE YOUR CHOLESTEROL LEVELS?
WRITE THEM IN THE APPROPRIATE BOXES BELOW:

RISK	LOW		BORDERLINE HIGH		HIGH	
	RANGE	MY SCORE	RANGE	MY SCORE	RANGE	MY SCORE
Total Cholesterol	<200		200-239		>or= 240	
LDL Cholesterol	<100		130-159		160-189	
HDL Cholesterol	> or=60				<40 in men <50 in women	
Triglycerides	<150		150-199		200-249	

SECTION 2 PRIMARY SESSION WELLNESS WORKSHEETS

as following a diet low in saturated fat and cholesterol, achieving and maintaining a desirable weight, and exercising regularly. The American Heart Association recommends that all adults age 20 or older have their cholesterol and other traditional risk factors checked every 4-6 years and work with their healthcare providers to determine their risk for cardiovascular disease and stroke.

6. High blood pressure increases the risk of heart attack and stroke. See the chart below for new blood pressure guidelines published by the American College of Cardiology and the American Heart Association in November 2017.

If your blood pressure is high or unusually low, talk to your doctor. Treatment and prevention for high blood pressure always involve lifestyle changes, such as weight control, increasing physical activity, and restriction of alcohol and sodium intake. An eating plan high in fruits and vegetables (3 ½ to 5 cups per day) and low-fat dairy products (2-3 cups per day) may also help.

WHAT IS YOUR BLOOD PRESSURE?

BLOOD PRESSURE CATEGORY	SYSTOLIC mm Hg (upper number)		DIATOLIC mm Hg (lower number)
NORMAL	less than 120	and	less than 80
ELEVATED	120 - 129	and	less than 80
HIGH BLOOD PRESSURE (HYPERTENSION) STAGE 1	130 - 139	or	80 - 89
HIGH BLOOD PRESSURE (HYPERTENSION) STAGE 2	140 or HIGHER	or	90 or HIGHER
HYPERTENSIVE CRISIS (consult your doctor immediately)	HIGHER than 180	and/or	HIGHER than 120
MY BLOOD PRESSURE			

MYplace **O** FOR NUTRITION

7. Physical inactivity. A sedentary lifestyle increases the risk of heart disease by nearly two times. This risk is as high as that caused by abnormal cholesterol levels, high blood pressure, *and* cigarette smoking combined! Despite the known risks, more than half of adults don't get enough physical activity to benefit their health. Regular moderate physical activity cuts your risk of dying from heart disease in half.

Are you getting at least 30 minutes of moderate physical activity several days each week?_____

8. Obesity and overweight. Excess body fat increases the risk for both heart attack and stroke. Obesity is also associated with increased blood pressure, abnormal cholesterol levels, and diabetes. Losing just 10% of excess weight and keeping it off can significantly lower your risk.

Are you within your healthy weight range? _____

9. Diabetes. Type 2 diabetes (high blood sugar) is very damaging to the heart and blood vessels. If you or a loved one has diabetes, it's important to do all you can to control blood sugar and other risk factors. A *fasting* blood sugar level of 100 to 125 mg/dl signals pre-diabetes, and a level greater than 125 mg/dl indicates diabetes.

What is your fasting blood sugar level?_____

10. Poor diet. This risk factor has been added to the list recently due to mounting nutrition research. A diet that's high in calories, saturated fats, sodium, and added sugars and low in essential nutrients contributes to poor heart health. (Yes, a steady diet of junk food is harmful—no surprise there, right?) In regard to sodium, some people are salt sensitive, meaning a high-salt (sodium) diet raises their high blood pressure; salt also keeps excess fluid in the body, which can add to the burden on the heart. On the other hand, making healthy food choices, such as fresh fruits/vegetables, whole grains, and healthy fats, more often can help lower blood pressure and improve heart health.

THE FACTS ON HEALTHY FATS

Risk factors 5, 6, 8 and 10 on the list above get a lot of attention in the nutrition world because making wise food choices can have a huge impact on them. One of the nutrition recommendations that all of these risk factors have in common is the recommendation to consume healthier fats as a way to improve the condition. So what is a healthy fat, and how much fat do you need to eat?

At one time, it was thought that a low-fat diet was a healthy eating style for everyone. Now, after hundreds of studies, we know that it's not so much the *amount* of fat as the *type* of fat that's important to heart health. You need an adequate amount of fat—about 45 to 75 grams per day on average—in your diet to help you absorb nutrients, increase your sense of fullness at meals, make your foods taste delicious, and promote optimal health and well-being.[8] The FP4H calorie levels are planned to meet these requirements, so when you follow your calorie level for the appropriate servings in each food group, especially focusing on the superfood choices, you will have no problem with this nutrient! It averages out to provide about 25-30% of your total calories.

The types of fats that you should be prioritizing in your diet to promote heart health are polyunsaturated fats (PUFAs) and monounsaturated fats (MUFAs). You need to *limit* saturated and trans fats.

SATURATED FATS are usually solid at room temperature and raise blood cholesterol levels more than any other type of fat. Animal foods such as meat, poultry, fish, butter, whole milk and cheese are high in saturated fats. One way that I remember this is thinking about the fat I drain off of my ground beef during cooking. What happens if you leave it out on the counter for any length of time? It hardens, right? This is a picture in my mind of the formation of fatty plaques in my arteries if I consume too much of this type of fat! Coconut oil and palm kernel oil are also high in saturated fat and should be limited just like animal fats. The American Heart Association recently recommended getting no more than 6% of your daily calories from saturated fat (about 13 grams per day for the average person). The FP4H plan is based on the most current USDA Dietary Guidelines that say no more than 10%—but lower is apparently even better!

TRANS FATS are also solid at room temperature and are usually chemically created through a process called "hydrogenation," turning a liquid vegetable oil into a bad fat (example: shortening). Trans fats do occur naturally in many foods, such as meat, butter, and milk, but these are consumed less than those produced by hydrogenation and are thought to be less dangerous than the artificial ones. Watch for the terms "hydrogenated _____oil" in product ingredient listings to know where this type of fat may show up, in addition to looking at the grams of trans fat on the nutrition facts label.

PUFAS (polyunsaturated fatty acids) are unsaturated fats found in nuts, seeds, and vegetable oils such as safflower, corn, sunflower, soybean, and cottonseed. Omega-3 fatty acids are a special type of PUFA linked with a range of health benefits, including heart and brain health.

MUFAS (monounsaturated fatty acids) are unsaturated fats found in avocados, peanut butter, nuts, seeds, olives, and vegetable oils such as canola, olive, peanut, and sunflower. (Many plant foods contain both PUFAs and MUFAs.) You may remember that olive oil is listed as a superfood in the Healthy Fats food group of the FP4H Live It plan. That is because current research links its use, especially in a Mediterranean-style eating pattern, with strong heart-healthy benefits.

It's important to keep in mind that fat (regardless of the source) is a concentrated source of energy, containing 9 calories per gram, compared to 4 calories per gram for protein and carbohydrates. Remember, just one teaspoon of oil contains about 40 calories. You don't need a lot of fat; just a teaspoon or two at each meal will get you the healthy fats you need without an over-abundance of calories. Too many calories from *any* source and not enough physical activity are the major challenges to weight management. Don't forget that you may be getting your one or two teaspoons of fat in the other foods you are already eating, so check your recipes and labels!

PREVENTING & MANAGING DIABETES

Diabetes is a group of diseases characterized by high blood sugar (glucose). If blood sugar builds up in the body and its levels are not controlled, it can lead to serious health complications, such as heart disease, stroke, kidney disease, blindness, amputations of the legs and feet, and early death. Diabetes was the seventh leading cause of death in the U.S. in 2010. Many people in my FP4H groups and some in my family have this disease, and you probably know someone with it also, since the most recent statistics reveal that 29.1 million people in the United States have diabetes. That's about 1 out of every 11 people! And 1 out of 4 of those do not even know they have it. Another 86 million people—more than 1 out of 3 adults—have prediabetes, and 9 out of 10 are not aware of that either.[x]

TYPE 1 DIABETES

This form of diabetes develops when the cells in the pancreas do not make enough insulin. This can occur at any age, but the peak ages for diagnosis are in the middle teen years. There is no known way to prevent type 1 diabetes. To survive, people with this type must have insulin delivered by injection or pump. Type 1 diabetes accounts for about 5% of all diagnosed cases of diabetes in U.S. adults.

TYPE 2 DIABETES

This form of diabetes is the most common, accounting for about 90-95% of diagnosed diabetes in U.S. adults. It usually begins as insulin resistance, a disorder in which cells, primarily within the muscles, liver, and fat tissue, do not use insulin properly. The risk of developing type 2 diabetes is associated with aging, obesity, family history of diabetes, a personal history of gestational diabetes (high blood sugar during pregnancy), not being physically active, race, and ethnicity. (There is a higher incidence of diabetes in Native Americans, Alaskan natives, African Americans and Hispanics than for Asian Americans or non-Hispanic whites.) Currently, it is projected that at least one 1 of 3 people will develop type 2 diabetes in their lifetime.

MYplace O FOR NUTRITION

PREDIABETES

People with prediabetes have blood sugar levels that are higher than normal but not high enough to be considered diabetes. Without weight loss and moderate physical activity, 15-30% of people with prediabetes will develop type 2 diabetes within 5 years.[9] There are no clear symptoms of prediabetes, so you may have it and not know it.

Symptoms of Diabetes

The following symptoms of diabetes are typical[10]. However, some people with type 2 diabetes have symptoms so mild that they go unnoticed:

- Urinating often

- Feeling very thirsty

- Feeling very hungry—even though you are eating

- Extreme fatigue

- Blurry vision

- Cuts/bruises that are slow to heal

- Weight loss—even though you are eating more (type 1)

- Tingling, pain or numbness in the hands/feet (type 2)

Early detection and treatment of diabetes can decrease the risk of developing the many complications of diabetes, so please see your doctor if you are exhibiting symptoms such as these.

Diagnosis of Diabetes

There are several ways to diagnose diabetes. Testing should be carried out in a health care setting.

1. A1C: This test measures your average blood glucose for the past 2-3 months; it does not require fasting. A normal A1C is less than 5.7%; prediabetes is 5.7 to 6.4%; and diabetes is diagnosed at an A1C of greater than or equal to 6.5%.

SECTION 2 **PRIMARY SESSION WELLNESS WORKSHEETS**

2. Fasting Plasma Glucose (FPG): This test checks your fasting blood glucose levels and is usually done first thing in the morning. A normal FPG is less than 100 mg/dl; prediabetes is 100-125 mg/dl; and diabetes is diagnosed when FPG is 126 mg/dl or higher.

3. Oral Glucose Tolerance Test (OGTT): This is a two-hour test that checks your blood glucose levels before and two hours after you drink a special sweet beverage. It tells the doctor how your body processes glucose. A normal OGTT is when the 2-hour glucose level is less than 140 mg/dl; prediabetes is 140-199 mg/dl; and diabetes is diagnosed when it is 200 mg/dl or higher.

Preventing Type 2 Diabetes

If your blood glucose is normal, take the healthy lifestyle steps that we advocate in FP4H to keep it that way, and undergo repeat testing every 3 years, or even more frequently if you are at a higher risk due to some of the factors listed above under "Type 2 Diabetes." If you have prediabetes, that does *not* mean that you will develop type 2 diabetes automatically! For some people with prediabetes, early treatment can actually return blood glucose levels to the normal range.

Research shows that you can lower your risk for type 2 diabetes by 58% by

o   Losing 7% of your body weight (or 15 pounds if you weigh 200 pounds)

o   Exercising moderately (such as brisk walking) 30 minutes a day, 5 days a week[11]

Management of Diabetes

The key components for diabetes management are (not surprisingly) incorporating a healthful eating pattern, regular physical activity, and pharmacotherapy (medications). If you are diagnosed with diabetes, your doctor will prescribe any needed medications and most likely refer you to a Registered Dietitian to help you determine an individualized eating plan to best manage your blood glucose levels, since there is no single eating pattern that is best for everyone with diabetes.[12] Most eating plans for diabetics involve carbohydrate-counting at some level, and some health experts also advocate using the Glycemic Index to assist with blood glucose control.

MYplace O FOR NUTRITION

Carb Counting

Carbohydrates (carbs) are naturally found in certain foods, such as grains, sweets, starchy vegetables, milk/yogurt, and fruits. When foods and drinks with carbohydrates are digested, the carbs break down into glucose to fuel our cells, and the body's blood glucose level rises. Carbohydrate counting assists type 1 diabetics with matching insulin doses to the grams of carbohydrate consumed at each meal/snack. Type 2 diabetics are often on oral medications to help manage glucose levels and are usually instructed to eat a consistent amount of carbohydrate at each meal throughout the day—not requiring quite the specifics of insulin-dependent diabetics. A common recommendation until an individualized plan can be determined is to eat three meals per day with about 45-60 grams of carbohydrate at each meal (or 3 to 4 carbohydrate choices, including whole grains, fruits, and fat-free/low-fat milk) with two snacks of 15-30 grams (or 1-2 choices).[13] One of my FP4H class members who has diabetes began eating breakfast each day, which she had never done, and found that it really did help her manage her blood sugar much better—*and* lose weight.

The Glycemic Index (GI)

The glycemic index measures how a carbohydrate-containing food raises blood glucose. Foods are ranked based on how they compare to a reference food—either glucose itself or white bread. A food with a high GI raises blood glucose more than a food with a medium or low GI. Meal planning with the GI involves choosing foods that have a low or medium GI; if eating a food with a high GI, you can combine it with low GI foods to help create balance. Examples of carbohydrate-containing foods with a low GI include dried beans and legumes, *all* non-starchy vegetables, some starchy vegetables like sweet potatoes, most fruit, and many whole-grain breads and cereals. Meats and fats don't have a GI because they do not contain carbohydrate. A few examples of really high GI foods are white bread, instant oatmeal, processed pasta mixes, saltine crackers, russet potatoes, and melons. Fat and fiber tend to lower the GI of a food, while cooking/higher processing tends to raise GI. When using the GI to assist with diabetes management, it is important to remember that portion sizes are still very important! Studies show that the total amount of carbohydrate in food, in general, is a stronger predictor of blood glu-

SECTION 2 PRIMARY SESSION WELLNESS WORKSHEETS

cose response than the GI. However, because the type of carbohydrate *can* affect blood glucose, using the GI may be helpful in fine-tuning blood glucose management. In other words, combined with carb counting, it may provide an additional benefit for achieving blood glucose goals for individuals who can and want to put extra effort into monitoring their food choices. If this interests you, just use your favorite Web search engine for more complete GI food listings.

Diabetes Superfoods

The American Diabetes Association has their own list of the top 10 superfoods. All of the foods in their list have a low GI and provide key nutrients: beans, dark/green leafy vegetables, citrus fruits, sweet potatoes, berries, tomatoes, fish high in Omega-3 fatty acids, whole grains, nuts, and fat-free milk/yogurt.[14] All of these are already noted as such in our FP4H Live It food plan lists.

Low Calorie/Artificial Sweeteners

When you have diabetes, including sugar-containing sweets in your diet is not taboo, but it does require careful planning since they contain relatively high amounts of carbohydrate. Foods and drinks that use artificial sweeteners (also called sugar substitutes, or non-nutritive sweeteners) are another option that may help curb your cravings for something sweet. They can be used to sweeten food and drinks for fewer calories and carbohydrate when they replace sugar. Between 1986 and 2010, the number of American adults eating and drinking sugar-free foods jumped from 78 million to 187 million, according to the Calorie Control Council. Diet soft drinks are the most popular sugar-free products.[15]

Even if you are not diabetic, you may ask, "Will artificial sweeteners help me lose weight?" Research reveals that 73% of people who consume low or no-calorie sweeteners say they use them to reduce their total daily calories. Products containing them may help with weight loss if they are used in place of their full-calorie counterparts—*provided you don't eat or drink those calories (or more!) through other sources.* Although the research isn't conclusive (in fact, it is rather controversial), some scientists believe that consuming food and beverages with artificial sweeteners can increase hunger, appetite, and calorie intake by decreasing the feeling of fullness or by training your taste buds to like sweet things so that you'll consume more of them. Obviously, the bottom line is that if you want the sweeteners to

MYplace ○ FOR NUTRITION

help you lose weight, don't eat more of something else to make up for the calories you saved.

It is also important to remember that, although artificial sweeteners can be used in place of sugar in many foods, thus lowering the calorie and carbohydrate content, this does not necessarily mean that those foods are carb-free, sugar-free, or calorie-free! When considering blood glucose and weight control, *be sure to check the nutrition facts labels for the total carbs and calories to make the best decisions.* Don't just go by the claims on the package that say "sugar-free," "reduced sugar," or "no sugar added," as some of these products actually have *more* calories and/or carbs than the regular versions.

There are currently six Food and Drug Administration (FDA)-approved artificial sweeteners and two "generally recognized as safe" (GRAS) artificial sweeteners in the United States. Based on current scientific evidence, the FDA has concluded that these meet the safety standard of "reasonable certainty of no harm" for the general population when they eat less than the acceptable daily intake. The American Academy of Nutrition and Dietetics (a professional association for Registered Dietitians) says that people can enjoy a range of nonnutritive sweeteners when they are part of an eating plan that is guided by current federal nutrition recommendations (such as the Dietary Guidelines for Americans, upon which the FP4H food plan is based) as well as individual health goals and personal preferences. The Academy does state, however, that there is not enough research on the safety of nonnutritive sweeteners during pregnancy or in the case of gestational diabetes.

See the "Know Your Sugar Substitutes" table on page 104 to learn how much of each sweetener you can eat and stay in the safe range:

Using Sugar Substitutes in the Kitchen

If you decide to use sugar substitutes when baking or cooking, there are a few important things to know:

- Baked products may be lighter in color because real sugar has a caramelizing/ browning effect and artificial sweeteners do not.

- Volume may be lower in cakes, muffins and quick breads because artificial sweeteners do not have the same bulking ability as sugar.

- Texture may be altered in some baked products, especially cookies.

- Taste may be slightly altered if you are sensitive to the sweetener's aftertaste.

- Cooking time of your baked goods may be slightly different when using artificial sweeteners. Sugar naturally holds in moisture and increases keeping quality so baked products with the sugar removed will not keep as long.

There are also some limitations of using sugar substitutes in food preparation:

- Aspartame is not a heat-stable sweetener, so it may not be the best choice when baking and cooking. When exposed to heat for a long period of time, it loses its sweet taste.

- Saccharin and sucralose are heat stable and are easiest to use in baking and cooking. However, to keep the desirable taste, volume, color and/or texture of a baked product, you usually will not substitute *all* of the sugar in a recipe for artificial sweetener.

- Read the package carefully for specific instructions on the best way to substitute the low-calorie sweetener for sugar in your recipes. The company's website can also be a helpful resource for baking tips.

MYplace O FOR NUTRITION

KNOW YOUR SUGAR SUBSTITUTES	Brand Name	Carb Grams Per Packet	Calories Per Packet	Number of Packets=to ADI*
Acesulfame K (Ace-K) if often combined with other sweeteners. It's about 200 times sweeter than sugar.	Sweet One Sunett	0	0	23
Advantame is 20,000 times sweeter than table sugar.	N/A	0	0	4920
Aspartame which is 200 times sweeter than sugar, shouldn't be used by people with the rare disease phenylketonuria (PKU).	Equal NutraSweet Sugar Twin	<1	0	75
Monk fruit, or Swingle fruit (Luo Han Guo), extract is GRAS**, but it's not regulated by the FDA as a food additive. It's about 150 to 200 times sweeter than sugar.	Monk Fruit in the Raw Nectresse PureFruit PureLo	<1	0	N/A
Neotame is 7000 to 13000 times sweeter than table sugar.	Newtame	0	0	23
Saccharin was first discovered and used in 1879. It has 200 to 700 times the sweetness of sugar.	Necta Sweet Sweet'N Low Sweet Twin	0.9	<4	45
Steviol glycosides (from the leaves of the stevia plant) include rebaudioside A, also known as reb A or Rebiana. They are GRAS** but are not regulated by the FDA as food additives. They're between 200 and 400 times sweeter than sugar.	Sweet Leaf PureVia Stevia in the Raw Truvia	0-1	<1-3	9
Sucralose which has 600 times the sweetness of sugar, works well in baked goods because it's heat stable.	Splenda	<1	0	23

*The number of packets a 132-pound person would need to consume to reach the acceptable daily intake (ADI).

** Generally recognized as safe.

"5 Must –Know Facts About Sweeteners," Diabetes Forecast (www.diabetesforecast.org), Meghann Moore, RD, CDE, author, January 2016.

SECTION 2 PRIMARY SESSION WELLNESS WORKSHEETS

DIABETES ACTIVITY

1. Do you have diabetes or have an increased risk for diabetes (based on the list under "Type 2 Diabetes")? _____
If so, when was the last time you had your fasting blood glucose tested, and what was the result? _____

_____

2. Calculate 7% of your current body weight: _____
Remember, just losing *this* amount and exercising at least 30 minutes, 5 days/week decreases your risk of advancing from prediabetes to type 2 diabetes by 58%!

3. Have you eaten any of the American Diabetic Association's superfoods this week, and if so, which ones? _____

_____

_____

_____

_____

4. Did you learn anything new about artificial sweeteners in this worksheet? If so, what? _____

_____

_____

_____

_____

JOIN THE SUPERFOODS FAN CLUB!

Do you like superheroes? I don't collect comic books or anything like that, but I guess I am what my daughter Kayla calls a "fangirl" at heart. I absolutely *love* to go and see the newest superhero movies, often wearing the corresponding T-shirt as I watch! My heart pounds, my hands grip the arms of the theater seat (and sometimes my husband Tony's arm), and I gasp when something crashes to the ground or flies at me (3-D, you know). I cheer as I watch them *always* defeat the bad guys with their daring and powerful moves, coming out seemingly unscathed from the battle! My personal favorites are Captain America and Superman (who will always be Christopher Reeve in my mind and heart), but there are many more that I love to watch as well. What makes superheroes super? They always have extra-special skills or strength, rising up above the regular people like me.

Most of my FP4H friends and group members would probably tell you that I am just as obsessed with superfoods as I am with superheroes, if not more so! New nutrition research is constantly being published now about the extra-special qualities in so many of the delicious and beautiful foods God has so lovingly created and provided for us on this earth. This research is showing that there are many foods that basically rise above others in the form of nutrition density and disease-fighting qualities, just like my movie superheroes rise above the norm. How exciting!

However, before we get into talking about individual foods, I must emphasize that what is *most* important in achieving a healthy body is *an overall healthy lifestyle*, which is what we teach in FP4H. Research shows that 80% of chronic diseases may be prevented simply by eating a balanced diet, getting regular exercise, avoiding tobacco, and limiting alcohol.

Let's begin our discussion of superfoods with a short biology lesson. The common roots of most chronic diseases are inflammation and oxidative stress. Short-term ("acute") inflammation is actually a good thing. This is our body's God-designed, natural response to an injury, such as when we get a cut on our finger. Our finger gets red, swollen, and painful as our body mounts a defense to ward off infection, and then returns to normal once the infection is resolved. But in long-term ("chronic") inflammation, the body's inflammatory reaction fails to shut off or possibly just becomes activated when there is no external trigger. This type of inflammation can go on for days, months, or even years; it may also be underlying, even below your pain threshold, so you don't know it is happening. Chronic inflammation of this type over time can become the foundation of many diseases.

Oxidative stress occurs when the level of free radicals in the body exceeds the capacity of the body's cells to detoxify these potentially harmful oxidants through its normal defense systems. Free radicals are formed by your body's own metabolism in day-to-day chemical reactions, but they also form as a response to environmental factors, such as radiation, toxins, tobacco, and pollution. Over time, oxidative stress can lead to diseases of aging. Antioxidants are like little sponges soaking up free radicals and helping to calm the immune system. Oxidative stress and inflammation go hand in hand—they can actually *cause* each other, making the situation worse and worse! One of the reasons that your diet has such a significant impact on your health is because substances in foods can help counter—or promote—these two conditions in your body. "Depending on your lifestyle choices, you can create an environment in your body that halts inflammation and oxidative stress in its tracks, or spurs it on."[16]

Studies have shown that diets high in refined starches and sugars, high in saturated/trans fats, low in whole plant foods, and low in fish appear to activate the body's inflammatory response. This dietary pattern is identified by nutrition researchers as the "Western diet"—an eating pattern found in industrialized nations, such as the U.S.—and has been associated with the development of many chronic diseases. However, a diet that is rich in whole plant foods, healthful carbohydrates and fats, and lean proteins cools down inflammation in the body. This wholesome eating pattern is what most of the major health organizations recommend and is the basis for the FP4H food plan, so you are on the right path!

Another eating pattern gaining a lot of attention is the Mediterranean-style diet, which is rich in fruits, vegetables, whole grains, nuts, beans, fish, and olive oil. A recent study showed that close adherence to this specific pattern can reduce heart disease risk by up to 47%. This study was comprised of 2,500 Greek adults, ages 18-89; participants who most closely followed this eating pattern over a 10-year period had the most benefit (American College of Cardiology's 64th Annual Scientific Session, 2015). With the flexibility of the FP4H plan, you can easily make Mediterranean-style choices in each food group to gain the same benefits.

MYplace O FOR NUTRITION

You can also fine-tune and enhance the disease-fighting attributes of your overall eating plan by frequently including the superfoods noted in each food group listing. Though there is still no technical definition for superfoods, these are foods that are packed with significant vitamins, minerals, and phytochemicals, which minimize the cell damage (inflammation/oxidation) discussed earlier. Others contain healthful fats, fiber, or amino acids that are protective against disease.

Most people have heard of vitamins and minerals and recognize them as being important to health, but *phytochemicals* may be a new term for you. These are plant compounds that serve as a natural defense system against environmental threats, such as sun damage, insects, pests, viruses, and drought. When I first learned about these, my thoughts went to Jesus' Sermon on the Mount, where He reminds us that our heavenly Father "clothes the grass of the fields" (Matthew 6:30). He took so much care in creating this world for us and sustains everything in nature so amazingly. Who knew that teeny little chemicals in plants could not only protect the plant but also protect *us* when we eat them? Phytochemicals have strong anti-inflammatory and antioxidant properties, enhance cell-to-cell communication in our bodies, cause cancer cells to die, repair DNA damage, and detoxify carcinogens (cancer-causing agents), just to name a few of their known beneficial actions.

Striving to eat a rainbow of fruits and vegetables (which are *all* superfoods) is a great first step in boosting your consumption of phytochemicals, because they are often the compounds that give plants color and/or flavor and are found in the plants' skin and flesh. Scientists have identified literally *thousands* of them, and new ones continue to be discovered. (Isn't God awesome?) Some very significant recent research also showed that the risk of death from all causes decreased 5% with each additional half cup serving of fruits and vegetables eaten each day up to a total of 5 servings—a potential 25% decreased risk! (See *British Medical Journal*, July 2014.)

SECTION 2 PRIMARY SESSION WELLNESS WORKSHEETS

The following are just a few specific superfoods highlighted in other recent studies:[17]

- Omega-3 fatty acids in fish can lower your risk of heart arrhythmias, lower levels of triglycerides and blood pressure, and slow the growth of plaque in your arteries. Other research shows that they may have other advantages: protection from inflammation, arthritis, depression, diabetes, and Alzheimer's disease. At the top of the Omega-3 fish list are shad, wild salmon, herring, sablefish, mackerel, whitefish (mixed species), and sardines.

- Consuming legumes (beans and peas) has been linked with lowering blood cholesterol levels and inflammation, reducing weight, and helping to prevent heart disease, high blood pressure, diabetes, and some types of cancer.

- In one cup, soybeans provide 57% of the Daily Value (DV) for protein, 41% DV of fiber, 49% DV of iron, and even 18% DV of calcium, besides a wide variety of phytochemicals! Eating soy has been linked to reducing cholesterol levels, lowering the risk of heart disease and prostate cancer, and may reduce hot flashes in menopausal women.

- Eating nuts regularly is linked with many benefits, including lower risk of heart disease, diabetes, metabolic syndrome, and some cancers. One recent study involving more than 70,000 adults showed that consistent nut and peanut intake reduced the risk of total mortality among U.S. participants by 21% (see *JAMA Internal Medicine*, 2015).

- Flax seeds contain unsaturated fats, Omega-3s, and are also very high in lignans (fiber compounds that act as powerful antioxidants) and mucilage (a type of gel-forming fiber that may improve absorption of nutrients in the body). Some recent studies have linked flax seed consumption with lower cholesterol levels (see *Journal of Nutrition*, April 2015).

- Studies show that eating oats daily lowers LDL (bad) cholesterol levels by 8-23%; they have also been found to increase feelings of fullness, lower blood pressure, lower fasting glucose levels, promote gastrointestinal function, and reduce the risk of type 2 diabetes.

MY place ○ FOR NUTRITION

- A diet high in whole grains (studies primarily included whole wheat) has been shown to reduce the risk of stroke by 30-36%, type 2 diabetes by 21-30%, and heart disease by 25-28%, as well as result in better weight maintenance and blood pressure.

- Barley (choose "hulled" or "hull-less" versus "pearled," which has some of the healthy bran/germ removed) has 8 grams of fiber in a half cup cooked serving, higher than most whole grains. Its documented health benefits include reduced blood pressure, blood glucose, and LDL (bad cholesterol) levels, plus increased feelings of fullness for weight control.

- The vibrant color in beets comes from the phytochemical beta-cyanin, which has been found to have anti-cancer effects. Beets are also a good source of dietary fiber, potassium, manganese, and vitamin C and also contain betaine, an amino acid shown to lower inflammation in the body. New research shows that beets may help fight heart disease by reducing LDL (bad) cholesterol and raising HDL (good) cholesterol, as well as reducing blood pressure.

- Literally *hundreds* of nutrition studies have been done involving broccoli! It provides high levels of vitamins A, C, and K, folic acid and fiber, as well as some protein and Omega-3 fatty acids. Findings include that it may reduce chronic inflammation/oxidative stress, which may ward off cancer; in addition, it may be helpful in promoting a healthy digestive system and good heart health.

- Carrots are very high in vitamin A (113% DV in a half cup) and have many phytochemicals linked to their vivid colors. Studies have linked carrot consumption to cardiovascular health, vision health, and cancer protection.

- Dark-green leafy vegetables, such as kale, spinach, collard greens, and chard are definitely nutrition superstars! They provide at least 19 essential nutrients in a one-cup (cooked) serving and have been linked to lots of health bonuses, including protection against age-related eye disease, cancer, osteoporosis, and even mental decline. A recent study whose findings were presented at the American Society for Nutrition's annual meeting revealed

SECTION 2 **PRIMARY SESSION WELLNESS WORKSHEETS**

that older adults (81+) who routinely ate 1-2 servings of leafy greens each day over a 5-year period demonstrated the mental capacity of someone more than a decade younger!

o Anthocyanins, phytochemicals in cherries, have been found to reduce arthritis symptoms, muscle pain, and the incidence of upper-respiratory symptoms after exercise.

o Studies place all types of berries at the top of the list in terms of antioxidant content and have identified that they have a profound impact on health, including lowering the risk of cancer, cardiovascular disease, diabetes, and age-related mental decline.

o Tea (all types) contains very high levels of phytochemicals in the form of flavonoids. Research suggests that tea consumption is linked with a lower risk of heart disease and certain cancers, protection of oral health, bone health, and immune function. To reap the most benefits, skip the pre-made teas and brew your own—the flavonoid contents of freshly brewed teas are much higher.

o Coffee—which contains over 1,000 active compounds with antioxidant properties—has been linked with improved mental and physical performance, a lower risk of type 2 diabetes, liver protection, and cancer-fighting properties.

And these are just a *few* of the studies! I hope this little taste will entice you to join the superfood fan club with me. Take a flying leap into the amazing, bountiful world of nutritious choices—you may never know what disease nemesis you may have battled and defeated until you get to heaven!

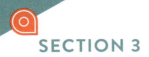

SECTION 3

Supplemental Wellness Worksheets

Fiber & Gluten Facts

Fiber is found *only* in the cell walls of plants—fruits, vegetables, and grains. Your body does not digest or absorb fiber, so it passes through your digestive system relatively intact. It is recommended that we eat 21-38 grams of fiber daily, from a combination of the two main types—*soluble* and *insoluble*.

SOLUBLE FIBER dissolves in water and forms a gel in the digestive system. The texture of foods such as cooked oatmeal comes from soluble fiber (just think of how it conforms to the shape of the bowl if it is allowed to cool completely). Soluble fiber lowers blood cholesterol levels by blocking the absorption of cholesterol and fats from the diet. Good sources of soluble fiber include oatmeal, barley, dried beans, peas, brown rice, and apples.

INSOLUBLE FIBER does *not* dissolve in water (think of bran flakes left in milk—no ge formed like the oatmeal mentioned above) and is more important to digestive health. It provides the roughage that improves bowel function and lowers your risk of colon cancer. Good sources of insoluble fibers are whole-grain breads and cereals, wheat bran, and most fruits and vegetables.

The importance of eating whole grains, a primary source of both types cf fiber in our diet, has been emphasized several times in this book thus far. But what makes

SECTION 3 SUPPLEMENTAL WELLNESS WORKSHEETS

them so special? A huge amount of scientific evidence links whole grains to a long list of health benefits, including:

o Decreased inflammation linked to chronic disease

o Protective effects against heart disease, stroke, and high blood pressure

o Protective effects against cancer and type 2 diabetes

o Reduced likelihood of being overweight or obese

o Reduced risk of developing gallstones, asthma, gum disease, and tooth loss

o Promotion of healthier carotid arteries

o Better gastrointestinal health

In fact, the proof of whole grain benefits is so strong that the U.S. Food and Drug Administration allows the following claim on whole-grain foods: "Diets rich in whole-grain foods and other plant foods, and low in saturated fat and cholesterol, may help reduce the risk of heart disease." A food must contain at least 51% whole grains and 11% fiber by weight to qualify for this health claim. As mentioned earlier in the "Grains" section of the food plan, the Dietary Guidelines recommend that all adults choose whole grains for at least *half* of the grains they eat every day.

5 Tips for Sifting Out Whole-Grain Products

1. At a minimum, look for whole grain to be listed first in the list of ingredients. Lots of breads and crackers contain whole grains, but if they're even second on the list, the product might contain as little as 1% whole grain!

2. Check out the fiber content. If a product provides only one or two grams per serving, chances are it doesn't contain much whole grain. Products that have at least 2.5-4.9 grams of fiber per serving are considered to be good sources, and foods offering 5 or more grams of fiber are considered excellent sources of fiber.

3. Don't be fooled by labels that boast "multi-grain" or "made with whole grain." Such wording is often actually a clue that the product is *not* 100% whole grain.

4. Look for "100% whole grain" on the front label; it means what it says.
5. Check the package label for one of two whole-grain stamps (see below), which can tell you if a product contains whole grains.

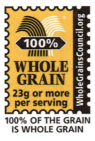
100% OF THE GRAIN IS WHOLE GRAIN

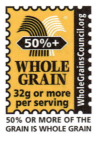
50% OR MORE OF THE GRAIN IS WHOLE GRAIN

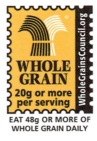
EAT 48g OR MORE OF WHOLE GRAIN DAILY

Be adventurous and don't restrict your diet to whole-grain breads and brown rice—there is a wide world of whole grains awaiting you that can offer unique health benefits and add flavor and texture to your diet. Try some amaranth, barley, buckwheat groats, bulgur, millet, oats, quinoa, teff, wheat berries and popcorn for variety. Just remember for popcorn that if you choose the microwave version, try to find one that is lower in fat (less than 4-5 grams per serving), lower in saturated fat (less than 1-2 grams), has zero trans fat, and is lower in sodium (less than 150 mg is best). And try your cereal grains both hot *and* cold—you might like one way much better than the other. Quinoa, for instance, is great in mixed hot dishes with stir-fried vegetables (my daughter Kayla loves to make a recipe called "California Quinoa" that has vegetables, feta cheese and calamari olives in it) or in cold salads with mixed dark greens, fruit and nuts (there's one at Panera Bread that I have enjoyed several times).

While eating more whole grains is recommended for *everyone*, some people get sick from certain grains, especially wheat (whole or refined), which contain gluten. An estimated 1 out of 133 people—two million Americans—suffer from celiac disease and must avoid all gluten-containing foods.[18] Celiac disease is an autoimmune disorder in which the body's immune system elicits an attack on the intestines when gluten is eaten.[19] Symptoms of this disease include diarrhea, gas, weight loss, anemia, bloating, fatigue, skin rashes, seizures and muscle cramps. While the symptoms

SECTION 3 **SUPPLEMENTAL WELLNESS WORKSHEETS**

are not *immediately* life-threatening, they can be quite debilitating. The first step to diagnosis of celiac disease involves a blood test to check for gluten antibodies. If you test positive, the next step is a biopsy of your small intestine to look for changes in the intestinal lining that are characteristic of the disease. Most intestinal damage is reversible if you follow a gluten-free diet, which excludes barley, rye and all varieties of wheat, including durum, semolina, spelt, triticale, and bulgur. Oats are OK to eat if they are certified gluten free; otherwise, they may be contaminated with wheat during growing or processing. Unlike food allergies that often disappear as you get older, celiac disease never goes away, and a gluten-free diet is a lifelong commitment, because continuous exposure to gluten can result in serious long-term health conditions, even for those who don't experience outward symptoms.

However, other people may have what is called "non-celiac gluten sensitivity" (also known as gluten sensitivity), which is *not* an autoimmune response—something different is going on in the body in response to the gluten. Symptoms often overlap with those of celiac disease and negatively affect quality of life, so physicians may recommend gluten restriction as a way to help decrease those symptoms. However, the intestines are not damaged and medical science doesn't know yet if there are long-term health consequences to eating gluten for people with this condition.

For best health, those with celiac disease or gluten-sensitivity still need to focus on getting at least half of their grains from gluten-free *whole* grains like brown rice, quinoa, and oats that are certified as gluten-free. For people with neither of those conditions, I would recommend that you eat a wide variety of whole grains, *including* whole wheat, due to the many studies that have shown its consumption as not only safe but also advantageous.

LIVE IT THE VEGETARIAN WAY

People choose vegetarian diets for many reasons, including personal preference, health concerns, dislike for meat or other food from animals, or the belief that a plant-based diet is healthier.[20] Others adopt a vegetarian lifestyle for ethical reasons.

Many people make the switch to a vegetarian diet simply because of the potential health benefits. Vegetarian eating patterns have been associated with improved health outcomes, including lower levels of obesity, a reduced risk of heart disease, and lower blood pressure. Also, vegetarians tend to consume a *lower* proportion of calories from fat, and fewer overall calories, and *more* fiber, potassium, and vitamin C than non-vegetarians.

There are many types of vegetarians. The following is a list of the most common variations:
1. Vegans are strict vegetarians who eat only plant foods such as fruits, vegetables, legumes (dried beans and peas), grains, seeds and nuts.
2. Lacto-vegetarians include cheese and other dairy products in their diet.
3. Lacto-ovo vegetarians include both eggs and dairy products.
4. Pescetarians include fish.
5. Semi-vegetarians exclude red meat but occasionally include poultry and fish.

Vegetarian diets can easily meet all of the FP4H recommendations for a balanced diet. The key is to consume a wide variety of foods and the right amount of food in each food group to meet your calorie goals for weight loss or maintenance, just like with diets that include meat. Specific nutrients that vegetarians may need to focus on a little more include protein, iron, calcium, zinc, and vitamin B12.[21]

PROTEIN has many important functions in the body and is essential for growth and maintenance. Protein needs can easily be met by eating a variety of plant-based foods. Combining different protein sources in the same meal is not necessary. Sources of protein for vegetarians and vegans include beans, nuts, nut

SECTION 3   SUPPLEMENTAL WELLNESS WORKSHEETS

butters, peas, and soy products (tofu, tempeh, veggie burgers). Milk products and eggs are also good protein sources for lacto-ovo vegetarians.

IRON functions primarily as a carrier of oxygen in the blood. Iron sources for vegetarians and vegans include iron-fortified breakfast cereals, spinach, kidney beans, black-eyed peas, lentils, turnip greens, molasses, whole-wheat breads, peas, and some dried fruits (dried apricots, prunes, raisins).

CALCIUM is used for building bones and teeth and in maintaining bone strength. Sources of calcium for vegetarians and vegans include calcium-fortified soy milk, calcium-fortified breakfast cereals and orange juice, tofu made with calcium sulfate, and some dark-green leafy vegetables (collard greens, turnip greens, bok choy, mustard greens). The amount of calcium that can be absorbed from these foods varies. Consuming enough plant foods to meet calcium needs may be unrealistic for many. Milk products are excellent calcium sources for lacto vegetarians. Calcium supplements are another potential source.

ZINC is necessary for many biochemical reactions and also helps the immune system function properly. Sources of zinc for vegetarians and vegans include many types of beans (white beans, kidney beans, and chickpeas), zinc-fortified breakfast cereals, wheat germ, and pumpkin seeds. Milk products are a zinc source for lacto-vegetarians.

VITAMIN B12 is found in animal products and some fortified foods. Sources of vitamin B12 for vegetarians include milk products, eggs, and foods that have been fortified with vitamin B12. These include breakfast cereals, soy milk, veggie burgers, and nutritional yeast.

Tips for Vegetarians

- Build meals around protein sources that are naturally low in fat, such as beans, lentils, and rice. Don't overload meals with high-fat cheeses to replace the meat.

MYplace O FOR NUTRITION

○ Calcium-fortified soy milk provides calcium in amounts similar to milk. It is usually low in fat and does not contain cholesterol.

○ Many foods that typically contain meat or poultry can be made vegetarian. This can increase vegetable intake and cut saturated fat and cholesterol intake. Consider:
   — pasta primavera or pasta with marinara or pesto sauce
   — veggie pizza
   — vegetable lasagna
   — tofu-vegetable stir fry
   — vegetable lo mein
   — vegetable kabobs
   — bean burritos or tacos

○ A variety of vegetarian products look (and may taste) like their non-vegetarian counterparts but are usually lower in saturated fat and contain no cholesterol.

   — For breakfast, try soy-based sausage patties or links.
   — Rather than hamburgers, try veggie burgers. A variety are available, made with soy beans, vegetables, and/or rice.
   — Add vegetarian meat substitutes to soups and stews to boost protein without adding saturated fat or cholesterol. These include tempeh (cultured soybeans with a chewy texture), tofu, or wheat gluten (seitan).
   — For barbecues, try veggie burgers, soy hot dogs, marinated tofu or tempeh, and veggie kabobs.
   — Make bean burgers, lentil burgers, or pita halves with falafel (spicy ground-chickpea patties).
   — Some restaurants offer soy options (texturized vegetable protein) as a substitute for meat and soy cheese as a substitute for regular cheese.

○ Most restaurants can accommodate vegetarian modifications to menu items by substituting meatless sauces, omitting meat from stir-fries, and adding vegetables or pasta in place of meat. These substitutions are more likely to be available at restaurants that make food to order.

○ Many Asian and Indian restaurants offer a varied selection of vegetarian dishes.

OUTSMARTING THE SNACK ATTACK

Why do we always think "unhealthy" or "junk food" when we think of snacks? Maybe it's because the snack aisle at the grocery store is filled with chips, cookies, candy bars, and soft drinks! It's not the practice of snacking that is bad, but the usual choices. The truth is that your body actually works best when it refuels every 4 hours or so, and the best way to do this is to eat three light, well-balanced meals and two or three healthy snacks. Snacking may even help you lose weight by taming your appetite and by preventing the tendency to overeat or make poor choices later in the day. Use snacks not only to satisfy hunger but also to boost your energy and help you reach your goal for a healthy weight. Snack time can actually be a great time to get in your daily servings of fruits, vegetables, whole grains, and dairy foods. Keep a supply of healthy snacks in convenient locations (car, purse, laptop or gym bag, work) and *plan* to have healthy snacks between meals. But don't forget to measure your portions and record the snacks on your Live It Tracker to stay within your calorie goals.

My friend Helen Baratta, Director of Development for First Place for Health, has lost over 100 pounds on the program and has a presentation that she does called "Simply Satisfying Snacks." She says that the best snack to eat is one that is low in calories, high in nutrition, and keeps you feeling full longer. The worst is one that's high in calories, low in nutritional value, and leaves you hungry for more. So, satisfying hunger ranks high. She also stresses that we need to prevent boredom with snacks. We get hungry for different types of foods and want a snack that meets that specific hunger. The following are some of her healthy recommendations for each type:

CRUNCHY: almonds, cashews, cocoa-covered almonds, Special K crackers, apple slices, and cut-up vegetables (such as celery, carrots, snap peas, bell peppers) with some type of nutritious dip or spread like hummus or Laughing Cow cheese wedges (the 35-calorie variety). Popcorn, since it is a whole grain, is a great choice as long as it is air-popped or reduced fat (like Skinny Pop or some type of light microwave popcorn).

CHEWY: dried fruits like mango, apricots, papaya, or apples

MYplace ○ FOR NUTRITION

JUICY: peaches, clementines, grape tomatoes, cantaloupe

SWEET: baked apples, grilled pineapple, or fruit/yogurt parfait

SAVORY: guacamole/salsa with a measured portion of baked tortilla chips, hummus with veggies, meat jerky (preferably without nitrates added), a wrap made with turkey breast and Joseph bread, celery sticks with turkey/lean ham and a Laughing Cow cheese wedge, olives, and string cheese

FILLING: celery with peanut butter, hummus with a whole-grain pita/pita chips, ½ cup oatmeal made with skim or almond milk, fruit smoothies made with milk, frozen berries and bananas, or even mini sandwiches made with thin whole-wheat bread or Joseph bread and one of the following fillings:

1. Laughing Cow cheese, strawberries or blueberries

2. Almond or peanut butter (1T) with ½ banana

3. Laughing Cow cheese and cucumber slices

HOT: baked apple with cinnamon (core a Granny Smith apple, put a sprinkling of brown sugar and a little margarine in the center, sprinkle the whole thing with cinnamon, and microwave, covered, for 3 minutes or until the apple is soft), or a cup of vegetable soup

COLD: frozen blueberries, pineapple, or grapes; Aldi's Fit & Active fudge bar; McDonald's small cone

"Taste and see that the Lord is good; blessed is the one who takes refuge in Him."

—Psalm 34:8, NIV

PREVENTING OSTEOPOROSIS

Osteoporosis, a weakening of the bones due to the loss of calcium and other minerals, is one of the most significant health problems in the United States. Millions of Americans—54 million to be exact—have low bone density or osteoporosis.[22] In fact, about one in two women and up to one in four men over the age of 50 will break a bone due to osteoporosis. The disease causes an estimated two million broken bones every year! It is sometimes called a "silent disease" because there may be few, if any, noticeable changes to your health to indicate that you even have it. The first indication of osteoporosis often is when a bone breaks. The spine, hip, and wrists are the most common sites for fractures.

Bones are not dry and dull as you may think—they are constantly under construction. Throughout your life, you constantly lose old bone while you make new bone. Children and teenagers form bone faster than they lose it. Their bones keep getting denser until they reach what experts call "peak bone mass," the point where you will have the greatest amount of bone you will ever have. Peak bone mass usually happens between the ages of 18 and 25. The more bone you have at the time of peak bone mass, the less likely you are to break a bone or get osteoporosis later in life. As you age you can lose more bone than you form. In midlife, bone loss usually speeds up in both men and women. For most women, bone loss increases after menopause, when estrogen levels drop sharply; in the first 5-7 years of menopause, women they can lose up to 20% or more of their bone density.

The good news is that it's never too late at *any* age to take steps to protect your bones. Whatever your age, the habits you adopt now can affect your bone health for the rest of your life. *Now* is the time to take action!

What can you do to protect your bones?

1. Get enough calcium and vitamin D and eat a well-balanced diet with plenty of fruits and vegetables.

2. Engage in regular exercise (especially weight-bearing/strengthening exercises—see *My Place for Fitness* book for more information.

3. Avoid smoking and limit alcohol consumption.

CALCIUM

Calcium, the major nutrient needed to form new bone cells, is vital for bone health. Bones and teeth store more than 99% of the calcium in your body. Calcium needs change at different states of life:

o Children aged 4-8 need at least 1,000 mg of calcium a day.

o Children aged 9-18 need at least 1,300 mg of calcium a day.

o Adults aged 19-50 need at least 1,000 mg of calcium a day.

o Women over age 50 and men over age 70 need at least 1,200 mg a day.[23]

Some calcium-rich foods include milk, yogurt, cheese, and calcium-fortified soy milk, cereal and fruit juices. Other good sources include almonds, canned salmon or sarcines with bones, and dark-green leafy vegetables.

Reading Food Labels—How Much Calcium Am I Getting?

To determine how much calcium is in a particular food, check the nutrition facts panel of the food label for the daily value (DV) of calcium. Food labels list calcium as a percentage of the DV. This amount is based on 1,000 mg of calcium per day. For example:

o 30% DV of calcium equals 300 mg (the amount in one cup of cow's milk).

o 20% DV of calcium equals 200 mg of calcium.

o 15% DV of calcium equals 150 mg of calcium.

Calcium Supplements

Calcium is best absorbed and utilized from food sources, but if you find it difficult to get enough calcium from your diet, you might want to consider taking calcium supplements. The amount of calcium you need from a supplement depends on the amount of calcium you get from food. Aim to get the recommended daily amount of calcium you need from food first and supplement only if needed to make up for any shortfall. The most common calcium supplements are *calcium carbonate* and *calcium citrate*. Calcium carbonate is less expensive but requires an acidic environment for absorption; therefore, taking it with a meal is usually recommended, since there is more gastric acid present in the stomach while you are eating. For people who take certain medicines that *decrease* gastric acid (such as Prilosec or Nexium for gastric reflux), calcium citrate, the more expensive calcium supplement, is usually the better choice. Regardless of which type is chosen, supplement absorption is optimal when taken as individual doses of 500 mg or less, because your body can only absorb so much calcium at a given time—anything past this is just flushed out of your system unused. Although yet unclear, some experts suggest that too much calcium, especially in supplements, can increase the risk of heart disease. The Institute of Medicine recommends that total calcium intake, from supplements and diet combined, should be no more than 2,500 mg daily for people younger than 50 and 2,000 mg daily for people older than 50.

VITAMIN D

Vitamin D is necessary for calcium absorption and also improves bone health in other ways. If you don't get enough vitamin D, you may lose bone, have lower bone density, and be more likely to break bones as you age. Your skin makes vitamin D from the ultraviolet light (UVB rays) in sunlight; your body is able to store the vitamin and use it later. The amount of vitamin D your skin makes depends on the time of day, the season, the latitude, one's skin pigmentation, and other factors. Depending on where you live, vitamin D production may decrease or be completely absent during the winter. Sunlight alone may not be a good source for you anyway if you're housebound or if you regularly use sunscreen or avoid the sun entirely because of the risk of skin cancer. Scientists don't yet know the optimal daily dose of vitamin D for each person, but a good starting point is 600-800 international units (IU) a day through food or supplements (800-1,000 IU if you are over 50).

Vitamin D is naturally available in only a few foods, including fatty fish such as wild-caught mackerel, salmon and tuna. Vitamin D is also added to milk and to some brands of other dairy products, orange juice, soy milk, and cereals. Check the food label to see if vitamin D has been added to a particular product. One 8-ounce serving of milk usually has 25% of the daily value (DV) of vitamin D. The DV is based on a total daily intake of 400 IU of vitamin D. So, a serving of milk with 25% of the DV of vitamin D contains 100 IU of the vitamin.

Vitamin D Supplements

For people without other sources of vitamin D and especially with limited sun exposure, a supplement may be needed. Most multivitamins contain between 600 and 800 IU; up to 4,000 IU per day is safe for most people. There are two different types of supplements: vitamin D-2 (ergocalciferol) and vitamin D-3 (cholecalciferol). Either one is fine to use.

SECTION 3 SUPPLEMENTAL WELLNESS WORKSHEETS

DIETING DANGERS & SUPPLEMENTS: 10 RED FLAGS OF JUNK SCIENCE

Doesn't it seem like everyone has advice on weight loss? Television commercials/infomercials, magazine advertisements, self-help or health sections of book stores, Facebook, not to mention your neighbors and friends—all of them offer solutions! Most people realize that not everything they see, hear or read is accurate on this topic, but how do you sift the facts from the fiction and hype? Before you spend your hard-earned money on products that promise fast and easy results, do yourself a favor and stop to evaluate if they are truly legitimate claims. Critically evaluate them using your knowledge of what you know a healthy diet looks like and what it really takes to lose weight.

Spoiler alert: There is no magic pill!

These 10 flags will hopefully help you critique and evaluate weight loss products and programs so that you can spot a scam.

1. **It promises a quick fix.** You've seen ads like this: "Lose 20 pounds in two weeks!" Face it, permanent weight loss takes time and effort to achieve and maintain. Products that *safely* and *effectively* produce lightning-fast weight loss just don't exist. Did you know that our bodies can only chemically break down two pounds of fat tissue per week? Any other loss is usually water, or possibly muscle, which is not what you want to lose! And lots of research shows that an average weight loss of 1-2 pounds per week is the safest and most effective way to take weight off and keep it off. That is what the FP4H food plan is designed to do, by the way.

2. **It sounds too good to be true.** "Apply this cream and watch the fat melt away!" Look for telltale words like "miraculous," "breakthrough" and "exclusive." When extravagant claims make the product sound too good to be true, just leave it on the shelf and keep moving.

3. **It excludes adopting a healthy diet and regular exercise.** "You'll never need to diet or exercise again!" The formula for weight loss is still the same as it has always been since God created us: Burn more calories than you consume. Unhealthy diets and no exercise can seriously compromise your health.

MY place O FOR NUTRITION

4. **Recommendations are based on a single (or really small) study.**
"A clinical study proved that…" Products and programs need to be tested many times, with significant numbers of people over long periods of time in order to be credible. Read the fine print to see exactly how many participants the study had and how long it lasted—you'd be surprised how many have tested something like 10 people for only a two-week duration. The study should also be published in a reputable medical or health-related, peer-reviewed journal—not just a tabloid newspaper or Facebook article.

5. **Simplistic conclusions are made from a complex study.** "Everyone will benefit from this product!" Results and conclusions from complex studies often include inherent limitations and biases as well as specific recommendations for specific groups of people (for instance, it may have included only women over 50, so results wouldn't necessarily apply to everyone until other populations were tested as well).

6. **Dramatic statements used to market the product are completely the opposite of recommendations made by reputable scientific organizations.** "Cut out all bread from your diet—there is no benefit from consuming whole-grain foods!" The Academy of Nutrition and Dietetics, American Medical Association, American Cancer Society and American Diabetes Association did not become pillars of health education, promotion and research without earning it. Hundreds of health professionals helped build these organizations and continue to pledge their membership by adopting their code of ethics and principles of practice. It is much wiser to heed the advice and findings of these groups than the frail claims of one "famous" person or for-profit company.

7. **Foods are divided into categories of "eat" and "never eat," or a major food group is removed completely.** "Only eat bad foods on the weekends!" "Cut out all carbs for the first 3 weeks." Or, "No one should ever eat dairy foods!" A single food or meal doesn't make or break a healthful eating pattern overall. Also, every food group plays a special role with regard to nutrition—*none* of them should be omitted!

8. **Recommendations are made to help sell a specific product/nutrition supplement.** "Speed up your weight loss with our specially formulated dietary supplement!" The bottom line is that supplements are highly over-used and a big money-maker. Most people don't need supplements if they eat a wide variety of healthy *foods*. The nutrients, vitamins, minerals and active compounds (such as antioxidants and phytochemicals) in foods are

SECTION 3 SUPPLEMENTAL WELLNESS WORKSHEETS

usually completely sufficient to deliver the nutrition you need and are also much better absorbed. However, if you fall into one of the following categories, it would be wise to consult with your physician regarding your need for supplements, especially if you have never discussed the topic with him/her:

a. You are on a restrictive diet, eating fewer than 1,600 calories per day.

b. You are an older adult (50+).

c. You are a vegetarian or vegan.

d. You are pregnant or a woman of child-bearing age.

e. You have a medical condition that limits your food choices.

f. You have osteoporosis, iron-deficiency anemia, or a digestive disorder.

9. Dire warnings of danger are included with the product or program regimen. "May cause heart palpitations, nervousness, and nausea." Why take a chance with something that is extremely risky to your body (God's temple) when your alternative—eating a healthy diet and exercising regularly—is exactly the opposite?

10. The person(s) endorsing or selling the product is not a credible health professional in good standing with others in the healthcare community. "This program is doctor approved!" Research the credentials of the person you are listening to. A white lab coat can be purchased by anyone.

RESOURCES FOR THE CONSCIENTIOUS CONSUMER

The Better Business Bureau: www.bbb.org

The Food and Drug Administration: www.fda.gov

The Federal Trade Commission: www.ftc.gov

MYplace ○ FOR NUTRITION

WEIGHT-LOSS MAINTENANCE

You've made it! You are at your goal weight—so now what? In a nutshell, keep doing what you've been doing! The new healthy habits you have learned following the First Place for Health Live It food plan and exercise components are still just as important. As long as you remain just as active as you have been during your weight-loss journey, you can usually move over a column (or two) on the calorie level chart and still maintain your weight. Adjust your calories slowly and routinely assess if you are maintaining your weight. Keep attending your FP4H group and encourage those who are still working to get where you are—several members in my group have been attending for over 20 years! The group continues to serve as an encouragement and accountability source for all of us, and we continue to learn more and more of God's Word through the Bible studies, helping us keep our focus on Christ and the *reason* we want to be healthy!

Below is a list of some of the behavioral characteristics of the members of the National Weight Control Registry, an ongoing project that tracks people who successfully lose weight and keep it off. Registry members have lost an average of 66 lbs. (ranges from 30 to 300 lbs.) and kept it off for 5.5 years (range of curation from 1 to 66 years!):

○ Most follow a lower calorie, low-fat diet (and keep a diary of what they eat).

○ 78% eat breakfast every day.

○ 75% weigh themselves at least once a week.

○ 62% watch less than 10 hours of TV per week.

○ 90% exercise, on average, about 1 hour per day, with the most frequently reported activity being walking.[24]

As you can easily see, the behaviors promoted in the FP4H program are right in line with what has seemed to work for all of these people. Be sure to share with others how you lost your weight, and Who helped you—what an awesome witnessing opportunity! May God continue to bless your healthy lifestyle efforts as you put Him at the top of your priority list and diligently seek His will for your life.

SECTION 3 SUPPLEMENTAL WELLNESS WORKSHEETS

Therefore, since we are surrounded by such a great cloud of witnesses, let us throw off everything that hinders and the sin that so easily entangles. And let us run with perseverance the race marked out for us, fixing our eyes on Jesus, the pioneer and perfecter of faith. For the joy set before him he endured the cross, scorning its shame, and sat down at the right hand of the throne of God.

—Hebrews 12:1-2, NIV

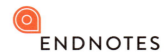

ENDNOTES

SECTION 1: THE LIVE-IT FOOD PLAN

[1] "Dietary References for Water, Potassium, Sodium, Chloride, and Sulfate," The National Academics, 2005, pages 86, 145-46.

SECTION 2: PRIMARY SESSION WELLNESS WORKSHEETS

[2] http://www.americanobesity.org/behavior.htm

[3] https://www.ucsfhealth.org/education/behavior_modification_ideas_for_weight_management

[4] United States Healthful Food Council, http://ushfc.org

[5] https://www.fda.gov/Food/GuidanceRegulation/GuidanceDocumentsRegulatoryinformation/LabelingNutrtion/ucm385663.htm

[6] http://www.cdc.gov/heartdisease/facts.htm

[7] www.heart.org

[8] "Superfoods: Eating for Optimum Health", a special report published by the editors of Environmental Nutrition, 2016, Sharon Palmer, RDN, author

[9] Centers for Disease Control and Prevention. Diabetes Report Card 2014. www.cdc.gov/diabetes/library/reports/congress.html

[10] American Diabetes Association, http://www.diabetes.org/diabetes-basics/symptoms, last edit April 1, 2016, accessed July 2016; also www.diabetes.org/diabetes/food-and-fitness.

[11] "The Role of Carbohydrates (CHOs) in the Management of Diabetes," www.eatrightpro.org, author Wendy Marcason, RD, October 2015, accessed July 2016.

[12] "The Role of Carbohydrates (CHOs) in the Management of Diabetes," www.eatrightpro.org, author Wendy Marcason, RD, October 2015, accessed July 2016.

[13] "The Basics of Carb Counting," www.diabetesforecast.org, author Allison Tsai, May 2015, accessed July 2016.

[14] American Diabetes Association, http://www.diabetes.org/diabetes-basics/symptoms, last edit April 1, 2016, accessed July 2016; also www.diabetes.org/diabetes/food-and-fitness.

[15] "5 Must-Know Facts About Sweeteners," Diabetes Forecast (www.diabetesforecast.org), Meghann Moore, RD, CDE, author, January 2016.

[16] "Superfoods: Eating for Optimum Health," a special report published by the editors of Environmental Nutrition, 2016, Sharon Palmer, RDN, author.

ENDNOTES

SECTION 3: SUPPLEMENTAL WELLNESS WORKSHEETS

[17] "Healthy Eating: Essential Strategies for Living a Longer and Healther Life," a special report published by the editors of Environmental Nutrition, 2014, Sharon Palmer, RD, author.

[18] "Healthy Eating: Essential Strategies for Living a Longer and Healther Life," a special report published by the editors of Environmental Nutrition, 2014, Sharon Palmer, RD, author.

[19] "Food Allergies, Celiac Disease and Gluten Sensitivity," www.eatright.org, published June 2015, Rachel Begun, MS, RDN, author"

[20] "Vegetarianism: The Basic Facts," www.eatright.org, published January 2016, Sharon Denny, MS, RDN, author

[21] "Tips for Vegetarians," www.choosemyplate.gov, last update July 2015, accessed July 2016.

[22] National Osteoporosis Foundation, http://www.nof.org/prevention

[23] "Understanding Osteoporosis," www.eatright.org, published May 2016, author Sharon Denney, MS, RDN

[24] https://www.ucsfhealth.org/education/behavior_modification_ideas_for_weight_management